To Ivy, Ronnie, and Ann
The Yin in the Yang

Acknowledgements

I wish to thank the many people who assisted me in creating this book. Master Henry Wang was, of course, the initial and persistent driving force. It was his idea from the start.

Master Raymond Chung, our first teacher, initiated my love for tai chi.

Diana Wood, taught me Mandarin, encouraged me to travel to Taiwan, and helped me understand Chinese culture. She has helped Henry adapt to life in Canada and still provides us tea before class.

Many of my students and fellow classmates encouraged me greatly. Beginning students, especially, were longing for a book that would specifically relate to Henry's concepts and which were unavailable elsewhere. More advanced students wanted more information about Henry's life and tai chi philosophy. Edgar Smith, one of Henry's advanced students, was instrumental in changing the format of the book from Henry's to mine. All the advanced students constantly provided feedback to further my tai chi skills and clarify my writing. Several students and friends provided photographs.

Ivy, Henry's wife, helped nourish me with food and emotional support.

Jan Lovewell helped me use my computer and did much of the initial editing. She and my wife, Ronnie, helped separate the wheat from the chaff, making the book more readable. Kim Boutilier has cheerfully been there to take my confusion of text, photos and calligraphy and put them into a presentable book. Ronnie has also continued to keep up my spirits when I felt the whole process too overwhelming. Even though this book depended on so many others, the responsibility for its contents is mine alone.

Song of Section I

I open my tai chi gate
I walking in a circle
I carry my good friend
We join together
I pet his back
And hold his hand
We swimming in the lake
I flow in the water
And touch the wave
I riding my horse
Across the field
I see the birds
Enjoying the sunshine
I see the crane
Stretch his wing
I walking my way
I enjoy my music
And play my pipa
I walking in my way
And see the people at the harvest time
I open my heart
And close my eyes
Enjoying my life
Flowing the tai chi way

MASTER HENRY WANG

In writing this book

I have deliberately chosen to spell

Chinese names in their most familiar

form. This may seem a bit confusing

to those who are used to Pinyin or

other accepted formats that translate

Chinese into English.

Also, for convenience, some words

such as "chi" and "tai chi" are select-

ed rather than "qi", ch'i, or "taiji."

Flowing
the Tai Chi Way

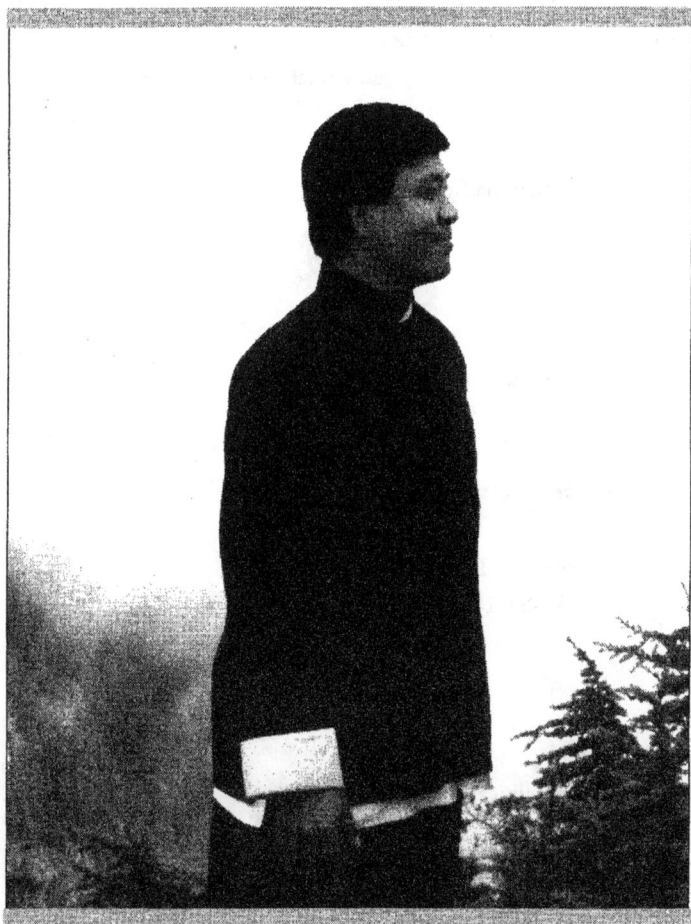

A Voyage of Discovery by a
Tai Chi Master and His Student

Peter Uhlmann, MD.

Peter Uhlmann, M.D.
Box 4, RR 2 Malaspina Rd.
Powell River, B.C. V8A 4Z3
Canada

Library of Congress Cataloguing
98-71807

Uhlmann, Peter, MD. – 1998

Flowing the Tai Chi Way
ISBN 0-8351-2636-6

Pinted and bound in Canada by
Navigator Communications

Introduction

Why write another book about tai chi? There are certainly plenty of books and magazines describing tai chi. Some are historical translations of Chinese texts on tai chi, martial arts, or Daoist philosophy. There are tai chi "classics" which describe traditional approaches, and are frequently quoted or referred to in reverential fashion. Similar to the Bible, these "classics" need to be interpreted since they are often written in a cryptic manner, and they can be difficult to understand unless the reader is familiar with Chinese culture and language.

There are also many "how to" books on tai chi. Each author will describe his or her particular style and form of tai chi and proceed to explain in great detail how to learn the art. Often there are many pages of photos, drawings, and diagrams to assist the reader in the learning process. Some books will coordinate a descriptive text with an accompanying video in which the author performs his/her form. I admire any student with the dedication and perseverance required to learn tai chi from a book or video, without regular lessons from a qualified teacher.

Other books describe a student's relationship with a famous tai chi master and often explain various aspects of the master's style and philosophy. These books may give insight into a tai chi practitioner's life and ideas, and they can make for enjoyable and enlightening reading.

Finally, there are books that go into significant "scientific" detail on tai chi as a martial art or as a path to improved health. There may be elaborate discussion on the nature of "chi" and its many forms and functions. Many people have described the health benefits gained by regular tai chi practice.

All the available literature on tai chi is valuable and serves various purposes. I must admit that it is difficult to advise beginning students, especially, on which books to read. Some are too detailed or esoteric for the new tai chi player and may discourage or confuse. Other books describe a form or style that differs significantly from what their teacher is promoting. For the more advanced students, the choices may be easier as they have some foundation in basic tai chi concepts and can select what new information is valuable to them.

Many tai chi students, and I include myself, look to books for "the secret" that will give them tai chi mastery, especially as a martial art, or in mobilizing and utilizing chi energy. Alas, though many authors claim to provide "the secret," I don't believe it is available in books.

I am reminded of the famous psychiatrist, Dr. Eric Berne. In one of his books he describes "the golden egg." He stated that patients in psychiatric therapy believed that their therapist possessed a "golden egg" which was a metaphor for the answers to all the patient's problems. If the patient came to treatment sessions on a regular basis and did all the right things, eventually the therapist would pull out the "golden egg" from his/her pocket and present it to the patient, who would then be cured. Of course, this never occurred, causing much frustration for both patient and therapist.

The study of tai chi can be similarly frustrating for the student and master since tai chi by its very nature is a life-long learning process and "never ending." There is no final "secret" or "cure." I find this quality of tai chi liberating. It means I can study and search for a lifetime and still continue to learn. I am suspicious of those who have final answers to any question, whether it be related to tai chi or any field of study.

So why am I adding to the tai chi library? Certainly I do not possess the definitive answers to all questions about tai chi. I am not a tai chi master and do not expect to achieve that position, nor am I an expert in Chinese culture or philosophy. I am an "unknown" on the greater tai chi stage.

I have studied tai chi for over a quarter century. For the past fifteen years I have had the privilege of a unique relationship with a tai chi master from Taiwan, now resident in Canada. I am also a medical doctor and psychiatrist with thirty years experience. I have some knowledge of physical and emotional health issues. I am also on a personal spiritual path though not specifically involved with an established religion.

Dr. Elizabeth Kubler-Ross has developed an interesting model to describe a person's health and development. She states people are composed of four quadrants. These are the physical, emotional, intellectual, and spiritual. For a person to enjoy good health, there must be healing and balance in these four areas. Tai chi has contributed to the ongoing development of my own quadrants. Initially I came to tai chi for the physical experience but soon realized significant emotional and intellectual benefits. I am only now appreciating tai chi's potential for spiritual progress.

In this book, I hope to convey my personal tai chi journey. Why was I initially attracted to tai chi, and why have I persevered all these years? What have I learned so far? What do I get out of it, and what more do I hope to achieve? How has tai chi contributed to and altered my life and my relationships? What is my relationship to my master?

This book is intended for several audiences. I hope that those of you who are attracted to tai chi, but have not yet become actively involved, are intrigued by the beauty and complexity of tai chi. I hope you will share my enthusiasm and find a place for tai chi in your life.

To tai chi players, I hope to share my process with you in hopes that your interest in tai chi will continue and your abilities increase. If you are not a student of my master, I hope you will keep an open mind and consider the value of his ideas. Often students become "stuck" or reach a plateau in their learning. I hope this book will allow you to continue your search.

Finally, for those students who have worked with my master, I have attempted to provide details of his principal concepts. I also hope to introduce him to you in a more personal way so that you can appreciate him as a person and not just as a tai chi master. He has been a powerful influence in my life, and I hope your experience will also be rewarding.

The Chinese say "A journey of a thousand miles starts with the first step." I am still on the tai chi journey, and this book is only a milestone. I sincerely hope that you, the reader will enjoy accompanying me along the path.

CENTRE

立身中正

CHAPTER ONE

Beginnings

One day in the fall of 1968, while walking our two Siberian huskies in New York's Riverside Park, my wife, Ronnie, and I happened upon an unfamiliar sight. Two men, one Chinese, were engaged in a back and forth dance. Though we did not know what they were doing, we stood fascinated by the beauty and energy in their movements. After watching them for a while, we continued our walk, storing the event in our memories. Years later I realized we were watching two players performing tai chi "push hands" exercises. I like to think that the Chinese man was the famous tai chi Grandmaster Cheng Man-Ching, who is primarily responsible for introducing tai chi to America, and who taught classes in New York during the sixties.

At that time Ronnie and I were in our late twenties and preparing to embark on travels through North Africa, Europe, and Asia. We spent a year abroad enjoying many freedoms and few responsibilities. It was the "hippie" era and a time of change in our lives. We were constantly exposed to different ideas and philosophies, and we tried to discover ourselves and the purpose of our lives. Like many of our peers, we experimented with drugs, encounter groups, yoga, meditation, eastern religions, communal living, and other counter culture concepts in hopes of arriving at some more enlightened place.

Two years later we were returning to California, where I had a licence to practice medicine, when we passed through Vancouver, British Columbia. Two friends we met on the island of Ibiza, Spain had invited us to stay with them in Vancouver. The combination of their hospitality, the unpleasant political situation in the United States, and the physical beauty of Vancouver convinced us to stay.

We found a charming house on the west side near the University of British Columbia, where I was accepted into a four-year residency training program in psychiatry. I began my studies, Ronnie was pregnant with our first child, and we began to feel settled for the first time in our seven years of marriage.

One evening Ronnie noticed an article in the weekend supplement of the local newspaper. The author described the activities of a Vancouver tai chi master. We remembered what we had witnessed in Riverside Park and we decided to phone the tai chi master and inquire about lessons.

The phone was answered by a Chinese man with a limited command of English. "You come my house 7:30!" he said. I tried in vain to get more specific information concerning cost, frequency, and content of lessons. All my questions received the same reply: "You come my house 7:30!"

Arriving shortly before 7:30, we entered the basement of an old house on Vancouver's east side. Several students, both Chinese and non-Chinese, were practicing tai chi, while a spry Chinese man in jogging pants and sneakers taught some individual students in a separate space. Master Raymond Chung was to become our first tai chi master. After finishing with the others, he took us aside and taught us the first movement in the tai chi form. He taught in the traditional manner. While he demonstrated a movement, we would observe and then try to copy him. He would make corrections and then send us home to practice until the next lesson. If we learned the movement to his satisfaction, he would teach us the next step. Because of Master Chung's limited English and our non-existent Chinese, there was minimal dialogue. We envied the Chinese students who would chat with him non-stop. Later we discovered they were not talking about tai chi. Even the Chinese students learned through the "observe-and-copy" method. It seems the conversations were purely social and often involved issues such as which restaurant to attend after tai chi class.

For over two years, we attended lessons twice a week. We learned one side of the Yang style long form with its 108 movements. Later we studied several methods of "push hands" and finally we studied "applications" with the ritualized offensive and defensive movements. Attending classes was similar to visiting a new family. We made many friends among the students, and Master Chung was like a friendly father. Tai chi became part of our lives, and we enjoyed the discipline of daily practice.

Ronnie became pregnant with our second child. At classes, Master Chung would tell her, "You have beautiful tai chi baby." When our daughter was born, we named her Tai.

We began to learn more about tai chi from the other students and by reading books. Tai chi was created thousands of years ago in China. Legends tell us that the ancient Chinese observed the animals in their environment and tried to copy their actions. Today many tai chi postures carry poetic names such as "monkey steps back," "golden cock stands on one leg," "white crane spreads its wings," "snake creeps down," etc. The individual movements were eventually connected in a sequential pattern, resulting in a tai chi "form," used initially for martial arts purposes. Many of the positions consist of punches, pulls, and kicks used originally for combat.

Over the centuries, tai chi changed and progressed. Many famous teachers emerged and passed their knowledge and secrets to their children or favourite students. Tai chi was studied primarily by the upper classes, who had the time and money to learn. Specific styles of tai chi developed and were named after the teachers who created them. Today we study tai chi styles that originated several hundred years ago. Many of the famous teachers are fifth or sixth generation descendants in their families. In North America the popular styles are named after their founders: Yang, Chen, Wu, and Sun. Grandmaster Cheng Man-Ching studied with the Yang family. He condensed the more than one hundred movements to thirty seven. Because of his martial skills he became famous in China and Taiwan. He was invited to teach in New York, and many present-day American teachers studied with him there. Like many tai chi masters, he was also proficient at skills such as calligraphy, acupuncture, art, and herbal medicine.

Today tai chi is popular around the world. Though tai chi is a martial art, it is primarily taught for its health benefits and stress reduction. The Chinese have had the opportunity to study health and disease for thousands of years. They believe in an energy called "chi." (This "chi" is not the same word as the "chi" in tai chi.) In Chinese medicine this "chi" is everywhere and can come into the body from the ground or sky. Illness implies a disturbance or imbalance of chi in the body. Some energy is "yang" or sun energy, while other energy is "yin" or shadow energy. Yin and yang should be in harmony and balance. Just as electricity requires a balance of positive and negative energy, chi requires a balance of yin and yang.

Chi circulates in the body similar to blood flowing through veins. Chi travels via meridians which connect with various organs in the body. Chi is stored in the "dan tien," which is located inside the pelvis below the navel. If chi flow is interrupted or imbalanced, then it can be corrected by Chinese herbs, dietary change, acupuncture, or other techniques of Chinese traditional medicine.

Tai chi is also a method for achieving health through proper circulation of chi. By practicing the form on a regular daily schedule chi is stored and balanced. This chi can also be utilized by skilled tai chi practitioners to heal others. Finally chi can be used in martial art applications for self defense. Tai chi is described as an internal fighting form since it depends on the use of chi energy rather than on the muscular strength which external forms utilize.

Presently tai chi is practiced by millions in China and around the world for health and relaxation. One can even learn about tai chi on the internet! After learning one or more form styles, students study push hands, which helps to develop sensitivity. Some students will learn tai chi weapons using swords, spears, or knives. The possibilities for tai chi study are really endless.

One translation for tai chi is "supreme ultimate." This implies infinite possibilities. Now as I look back at our tai chi lessons with Master Chung, I realize we were just floating on the surface of an ocean of potential. We had learned some movements and put them into a dance-like pattern. We practiced push hands with little appreciation of the underlying dynamics involved. This was not the fault of our teacher. We had not yet developed the maturity and experience to understand tai chi.

Also, our lives had limited time for tai chi. I was studying psychiatry and working full time at a job that was physically and emotionally demanding. As well we had two small daughters, and parenting was our top priority. It's not easy to get up early and practice form when you are exhausted from work and child care. Children don't understand parents wanting some time for personal pursuits. Many times I practiced a new movement called "shaking small child from leg"!

Finally, after two years in Vancouver, we moved to Powell River, British Columbia, a small, isolated mill town on the coast. Though we were only eighty miles from Vancouver as the crow flies, the drive required five hours travel, including two ferry trips. Our continued attendance at Master Chung's tai chi class steadily decreased. Without the stimulation of his class and the other students, we eventually discontinued our tai chi practice. We kept occasional contact with Master Chung and tried to attend the yearly tai chi banquet. This was a grand affair at a downtown Chinese restaurant. Aside from the food and drink, students would demonstrate their skills. Master Chung would provide us with a rare performance of other internal martial arts related to tai chi.

In 1978, I had the opportunity to visit mainland China with a group of medical workers. I spent two weeks travelling through China at a time when visitors were still a novelty. In Shanghai I awoke early and watched hundreds of Chinese practicing tai chi by the river. I was told that only older people liked tai chi and that modern Chinese youth preferred jogging.

In Guangzhou I made contact with Master Chung's wife and daughter. This was not easy to arrange, but I persisted. They came for a brief visit to my hotel and presented me with gifts of a lace tablecloth and a picture painted by the daughter. They also gave me some herbs to bring home to Master Chung. I was amazed when Canada Customs allowed me through with them.

Master Chung had been separated for seventeen years from his wife and two children. He had been in Hong Kong with two older daughters when the Communists closed the border, blocking his return. He emigrated to Canada with the two girls. In Vancouver he supported his two daughters and sent extra funds to the rest of his family in China. Happily his wife and children were reunited with him six months after my visit to Guangzhou. Today his wife and son are also tai chi teachers.

The trip through China stimulated me to study Mandarin Chinese. Diana, a Powell River friend, was raised in Taiwan and became my teacher. Eventually I wanted to live in a Chinese culture and improve my language skills, but mainland China presented too many obstacles. Taiwan, on the other hand, encouraged foreign students to study Mandarin. In December, 1982, our family travelled to Taipei, the capital of Taiwan, and I enrolled at the Mandarin Training Centre. We found an apartment and began to experience Chinese culture in earnest. Ronnie taught English. Our two daughters attended Taiwanese elementary school, while Sasha, our five-year-old son, attended preschool. While in Taipei, we decided to find a tai chi teacher and renew our studies.

RELAXATION

全身放鬆

CHAPTER TWO

Meeting Our Master

It had been ten years since we studied tai chi. We had been working on our emotional and intellectual quadrants, and paying less attention to our physical and spiritual needs. I have never been able to predict the course of my life. My father was a physician, and there were certainly expectations that I would follow in his footsteps. I struggled through my pre-med courses and preferred liberal arts, but when I entered medical school I found I actually enjoyed it. Medicine has been very good to me, and I feel I have made my contributions as well; however, there has always been a part of me that wished I had chosen a different path. I have always felt a stranger in my own land, which may explain why I have been attracted to other cultures. In college I studied Russian language and history, with a view to serving overseas in the diplomatic corps, but I chose medicine as "more practical." How different my life might have been.

My family were Jews who left Germany in the thirties to escape the Holocaust. We spoke German at home, and this contributed to my interest in languages. I have only recently come to realize how the war in Europe affected my life growing up in America. My family never spoke of the horror they experienced, yet the unconscious messages were there for me to receive. Feelings of sadness and separateness were some of the consequences of the Holocaust for me. Because they were unconscious, I was unaware until recently how they determined many of my behaviours and choices. One of these choices was the strong need to be in control of my life and environment. This need to be in control has taken its toll, and stress is one result. For me, tai chi offered relief from tension and stress and an opportunity to learn how to relax and "let go." "Letting go" became a major theme in my life, and it continues to be one today.

So here we were in Taipei, Taiwan. I "let go" of my medical practice in Powell River for a year, and we took the kids out of school for a different type of education. Taiwan in 1982 still retained some of the charm of traditional China. It felt safe to walk about, people were very friendly, and food was cheap and of excellent quality. The down side was crowds, traffic, and pollution. We began to learn Chinese language and traditions. The latter were most important. For example, our landlord took it upon himself to be responsible for us while we lived in his apartment. This meant inviting us to his home or out into the community to visit or dine. We could not return any of his generosity as that would have been insulting. On the other hand, he told us he would expect the same care should he visit us in Canada (which he never did).

Chinese have a concept of "guanxi" (pronounced guan shee). This means relationships or connections. To get things done requires guanxi. This is similar to our "It's not what you know. It's who you know." You scratch my back, and I'll scratch yours. Guanxi is seen in a positive light, and this is important. It did take us a while to get used to. Furthermore, once guanxi relationships are established, they can be life long. Therefore, one is initially cautious about committing oneself.

How does this relate to tai chi? To find a tai chi master and be accepted as a student requires guanxi among other things. In Canada if I want to study something, I find the course, pay my money, and expect the teacher to satisfy my needs. Not so for a tai chi master! First there must be proper introductions through an intermediary, then proper respect must be shown to the master, after which he may or may not decide to accept a pupil. Then the student is expected to please the master, not vice versa. Once accepted by a master, the relationship is for life. Even if one leaves or changes masters, the respect for the first master never ends.

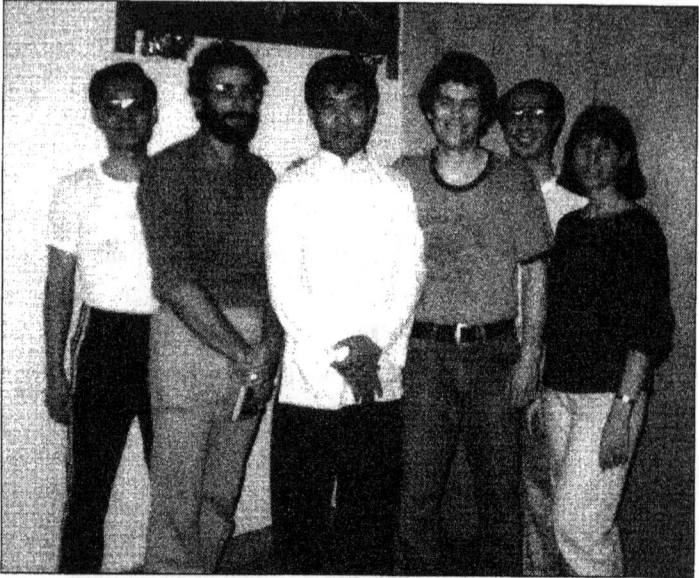

The author (second from left) and Ronnie (far right) attending tai chi class at Master Wangs home in Taipei, Taiwan, 1983.

Teachers are highly revered in Chinese culture. Only one's parents receive more respect. Students follow the teacher's instructions to the letter and don't question the teacher's authority. How different from the West, where teachers encourage questions from their students. To ask a question of a Chinese teacher is insulting and implies they have not taught properly. Our daughter, Tanya, was in a Taiwanese elementary school and was asked to draw a tree in art class. First the teacher drew a tree on the blackboard for the students to see. Tanya cheerfully engaged herself in drawing a tree. The teacher came around to her desk and was horrified to see that she was not copying his tree from the blackboard like the other students. It was not easy to explain to Tanya the different expectations in Taiwan and Canada.

Prior to leaving Canada, I had approached a psychiatrist at UBC who originally came from Taiwan. He gave me the names and addresses of some close friends in Taiwan who could offer us assistance. This was a good example of guanxi. These friends connected us to a couple from Australia who lived in Taipei. The husband, originally from the States, was fluent in Chinese. He worked as an anthropologist and was able to teach us a lot about Taiwan. His wife was originally from Hong Kong. She was interested in many martial arts and had studied tai chi. We asked her if she could arrange tai chi instruction for us. She told us the best tai chi master in Taiwan was Master Wang Hui-Juin, or Henry Wang.

After making some inquiries, our friend arranged an introductory meeting with Master Wang. He had a regular day-time job at a fitness centre in Taipei. Teaching tai chi had not yet become his sole source of income. His reputation as a tai chi master was growing, and he had accepted a few students who went to his home to study. He lived in the basement suite of an apartment building with storefronts on the street level. One of these was his teaching studio. When we arrived with our friend, Master Wang was teaching some of his other pupils. He was very friendly and warm. He seemed genuinely interested in meeting us and preferred to practice his rudimentary English rather than listen to my crude Mandarin.

Master Wang asked Ronnie and me to demonstrate the tai chi form we had studied in Vancouver. Though we felt rusty, we performed the form to the best of our ability. I think we even hoped we might impress him and receive some compliments. Instead he commented, "Very pretty, but empty." We somewhat resentfully asked what he meant by "empty." He didn't speak, but instead proceeded to demonstrate his form. When he had finished, we understood! Our tai chi movements were graceful and dance-like, but lacked substance, lacked "chi." Watching Master Wang we could feel an energy coming from him while he moved through the tai chi postures. We were in the presence of a master with exceptional skill, and moreover he agreed to accept us as his students. We made the necessary arrangements regarding time and cost of lessons, settling on two evenings a week. We left his studio with our friend, whom we thanked, and went home.

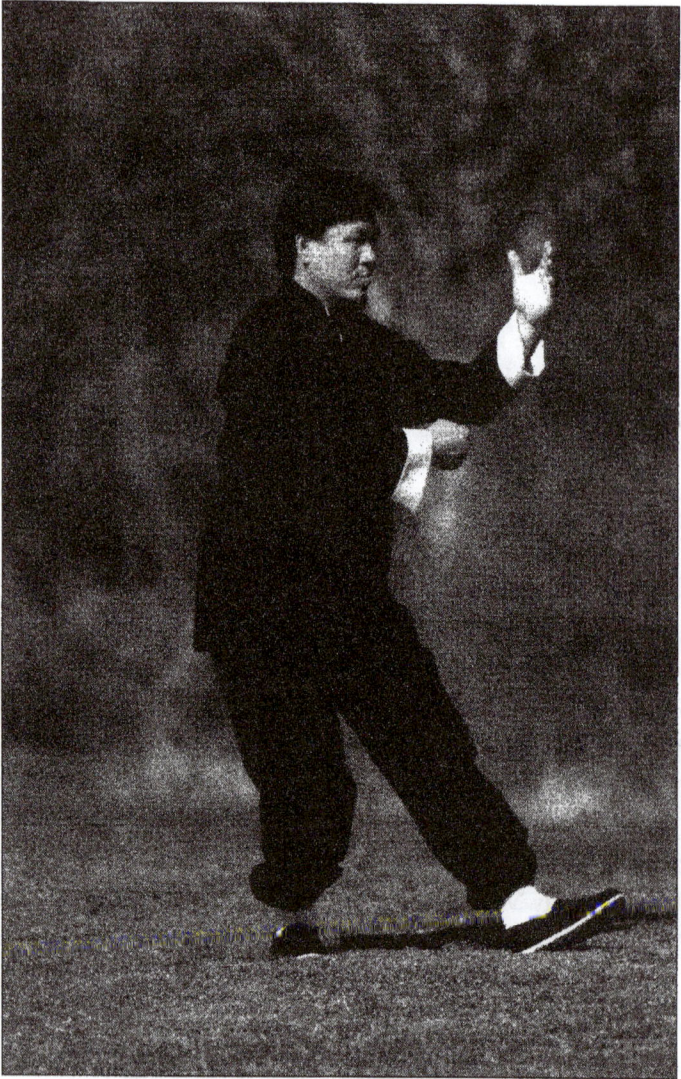

Henry demonstrating tai chi posture "Right Fist Under Elbow."

At this point I wish to take the liberty of referring to Master Wang as Henry, for the rest of the book. This is not just for convenience though that is a factor. As I implied above, the title of teacher or master in China is extremely important. However, it will become obvious to you, the reader, that my relationship with Henry developed into much more than master-pupil. In tai chi class or any learning situation, I always address Henry as Master Wang or "Shirfu," the Chinese word for Master. Outside class he is always Henry. Unlike many Chinese teachers and masters, Henry remains friendly and approachable to his students and friends. Because of this unique quality of his, he is comfortable being called Henry. My great respect for him as a master and friend is not influenced by his title.

When we started our studies, Henry tried to improve our form, but it became mutually apparent that we had to start over from the beginning. Even more difficult was unlearning some of the bad habits we had acquired over the years. It was very humbling to realize how little we knew despite years of effort. Because we would only be in Taiwan for four more months, he concentrated on teaching us his approach to some of the more familiar tai chi postures. We would then put them together in some sequence to form a short pattern. The concept that we could alter and play with the tai chi postures was a new one for us. He also showed us some exercises to help us relax our backs and shoulders. We looked forward to our classes and enjoyed meeting the other students. We also saw Henry "push hands" with some of his more advanced students, often sending them flying backwards until stopped by the wall or another pupil. His martial art skills were exciting to watch, and he would occasionally demonstrate on us.

At this point in our relationship, Henry was our master, but we had no social interaction. We met Ivy, his wife, and their two children, but only to say hello. We had to travel almost an hour each way on very crowded buses to attend classes, and the pace of life in Taiwan left little time for entertaining. He told us about other foreign students who had studied with him briefly, and how he hoped eventually to travel abroad and visit them. Ronnie asked Henry if he would consider moving to Powell River to teach tai chi. To my surprise he indicated considerable interest. We told him we would research the possibilities when we returned to Canada. Our four months of lessons went by quickly. For our final class we invited Henry's family to a nearby restaurant for a farewell dinner. We realized then that we had become close, and it was sad to say good bye.

Our family left Taiwan to continue our travels through Hong Kong, Mainland China, Russia, India, and Thailand, returning just before New Years, 1984. Again we allowed our busy lives to be in control while tai chi practice took a back seat. It seems we needed the regular presence of a teacher to keep us on track.

CHAPTER THREE

Henry Wang

Who was this tai chi master who entered our lives and would soon become a major influence? Despite many years of close friendship, I know only a few details of Henry's life. Personal disclosure is not a common Chinese trait. Many years ago, I read the autobiography of Dr. Carl Jung, the famous Swiss psychoanalyst. His book focused on his thoughts, dreams, and work. There was almost nothing about his personal life. Similarly, Henry shares information about his life as it directly relates to tai chi. He won't even tell me his birth date. What he has shared gives some insight into his choice of tai chi as a life's path.

Henry was born in 1951, in Taiwan, and lived there until immigrating to Canada in 1987. He is the eldest of three boys. His father left mainland China after the war and married Henry's mother, who was from Taiwan. As a child Henry's physical health was impaired as he suffered from asthma. He remembers having difficulty breathing in elementary school and being unable to participate in strenuous sports. He was shy and embarrassed to stand in front of the class and read aloud. He lacked self confidence.

He was not interested in academics, which can be a real handicap in Chinese society with its great emphasis on performing well in school. He recalled feeling different from his classmates in that he did not share their interest in clothes and other material things. He enjoyed nature and was curious about people, ideas, and spiritual issues. He was not raised in any formal faith, but in Taiwan there are many traditional concepts and temples.

Taiwanese parents place incredible pressure on their children to succeed in school and work. "A good student has a good future." Often when Ronnie and I rode the late night bus back home from our tai chi lesson, we would share the seats with exhausted students who were attending night school "cram" courses. This was in addition to their regular schooling. We felt sorry for these kids, who weren't allowed much of a childhood.

Chinese children learn to obey and respect their family, a concept known as "filial piety." Henry loved his family but felt he was not fulfilling their expectations of an eldest son.

He told me his first memory of tai chi was watching his own father practice, but as a child this provoked minimal interest. At age fourteen Henry began to study gymnastics. Since few Taiwanese were interested in that sport, he became a leader and with practice began to excel. He paid increased attention to his physical condition. As a result he gained in strength and confidence.

Around the age of sixteen, he became interested in gung fu. This coincided with the era of Bruce Lee and was quite fashionable. Gymnastics and martial arts became his major focus in life at that time. He practiced judo and shaolin boxing with dedication seven days a week.

When his high school days were over, he decided against attending university, which disappointed his family. They did not appreciate his devotion to sports and worried about Henry's future. He joined the army at age twenty, an obligation for all Taiwanese males. For the next two years he studied martial arts and became an army instructor. He says the army taught him to feel comfortable teaching in front of a group. He taught gung fu and tae kwon do. He found the army stressful and confining. He resented the lack of freedom and did not enjoy following orders. He disagreed with the army's philosophy of force to solve conflicts. He also realized he suffered from a quick temper.

After the army, he was undecided about his future. It was hard to find decent work without a college diploma. He attended journalism college for three years but lacked real motivation. At age twenty two he met Ivy, an art student and his future wife. They were married a year later. He found work with a construction company.

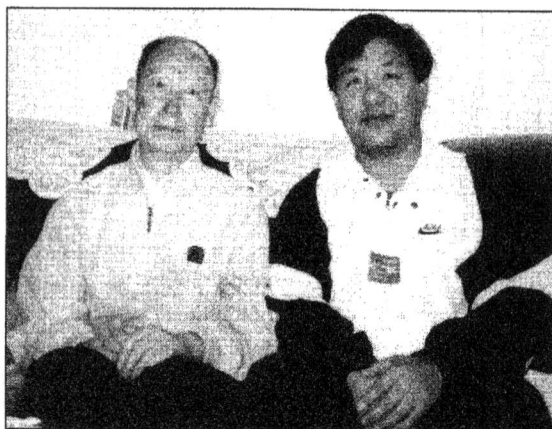

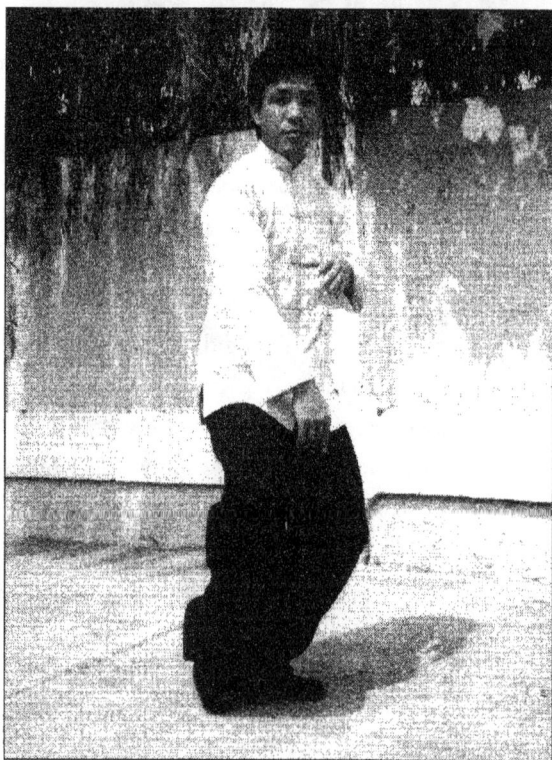

TOP: *Master Chang, Henry's philosophy teacher, and Henry in Taiwan.*
BOTTOM: *Early photo of Henry practicing in Taiwan.*

At twenty three Henry also began to study tai chi. He began to observe tai chi players in the Taipei parks. In China martial artists of all kinds gather in public parks to practice, study and compete with others. He seemed primarily interested in tai chi's reputed ability to soften one's temper. He chose to study Kwun Lun style tai chi and later the Yang style long form.

Henry was to learn from many different teachers. One of his first teachers, Kwun Lun-Pai, came from his father's home province of Hebei. Another teacher was Master Yang Yu-Jen, who eventually became chairman of the Taiwan Tai Chi Association. Later he studied with Master Chiang, the secretary of the Taipei Tai Chi Association. After one and a half years, Master Chiang urged Henry to enter a push hands competition. At age twenty five Henry entered and won the North Taiwan competition. Because of his excellent physical condition, he found the event easy to win. After the competition his body was sore for a week, and he realized how much force had been involved in defeating his opponents. His study of tai chi philosophy claimed that four ounces could move a thousand pounds, and that soft could triumph over hard. These concepts were obviously absent in the push hands competition.

The following year Henry met Master Chang, a professor of philosophy at Wen Hua University in Taiwan. Together they discussed tai chi and Daoist philosophy, especially the ideas of the ancient Chinese philosopher, Lao Tze. Master Chang has remained Henry's philosophy mentor to the present day. Chang also studied tai chi and had known Grandmaster Cheng Man-Ching. During their push hands practice together, Chang advised Henry to relax and become softer. Henry initially found this difficult.

Henry's ability improved under Chang's tutelage, and he placed second in a competition in Tai Chung. Nevertheless, Chang told him he was still too hard. Because of his success in competition, Henry attracted other tai chi students who wanted to practice with him. He practiced "neutralizing" by avoiding his opponent's pushes. This required him to relax and be softer. At his third push hands competition, an international event in Taipei, he won first place. He devoted all his spare time to the study of tai chi and its many styles.

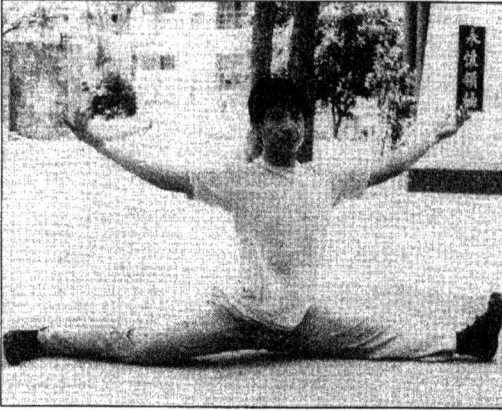

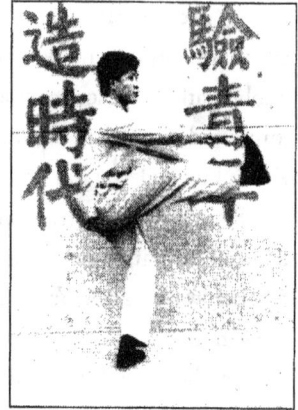

Early photos of Henry practicing in Taiwan.

Because he was away from home so much, his wife, Ivy, complained. By this time they had started a family, and the main responsibility for the children was hers. Because tai chi was viewed as a hobby or pastime, it was understandable that she resented the time he spent practicing. In her view, only a lucrative job deserved such time and effort.

A major turning point for Henry occurred during the 1980 international competition, which he won. Grandmaster Huang Sheng-Shyan from Malaysia and some of his senior students were present. Huang gave a demonstration of his tai chi skills, and Henry was very impressed. He wanted to study with Huang, but this was easier said than done. Every tai chi group kept their "secrets" well guarded, and teachers could only be contacted through their students. Though Huang was seventy years old at the time, Henry had never encountered a master with such ability. Through "guanxi" he was finally introduced to Huang. Huang was also curious about Henry, who had defeated Huang's student in the competition.

Henry made it his goal to be in the presence of Huang as much as possible. Each time Huang came to Taiwan, Henry was in attendance. He would arise early in the morning to serve Huang's needs. He would bring Huang his favourite foods and serve him as his disciple. He even had to learn a new

Chinese dialect as Huang did not speak proper Mandarin. This devotion to the master is traditional in Chinese culture.

During Huang's demonstrations, Henry observed a lot of power. He wondered how this power came through softness. Eventually one morning he went to Huang's hotel to practice with the students, and the Grandmaster let him practice push hands with him. Henry said he knew the second he touched Huang that he possessed the qualities Henry had been searching for. "He felt powerful, like a spring, but very soft." He realized that he had a lot more to learn even after winning several competitions. Huang emphasized softness and "investment in loss". This meant letting go of one's ego and experiencing progress by losing. (I'll return to this concept in a later chapter.) Henry continued to observe Huang and pick up any clues about his ability. He noted that none of Huang's students was nearly as skilled as their master.

After winning his fifth and final competition in 1981, Henry became a "target" for many martial art students wanting to test their skills against a champion. Henry wanted to prove to himself that tai chi was the ultimate martial art and that softness could overcome hardness. Therefore he initially enjoyed the challenges. One unfortunate incident occurred when he was set up to practice with a large American in a Taipei park. At first all was friendly between them, but the American became increasingly frustrated when he couldn't defeat Henry. The American made a sudden aggressive move which Henry neutralized, but the American broke his own arm in the process. Later he tried to sue Henry for financial compensation, but Henry's own students chose to settle the matter out of court, saving Henry any further hassle. This experience taught Henry to be more cautious and to limit his further practice with his own students. He realized there was no limit to the number of fighters who would want to challenge him, and it would prove nothing if he engaged them all.

Henry had been feeling his prospects in Taiwan were limited. Earning a living was stressful, despite working in a fitness centre. He felt the environment there was not conducive to his advancement in tai chi. He was open to other life options when we met him in 1983.

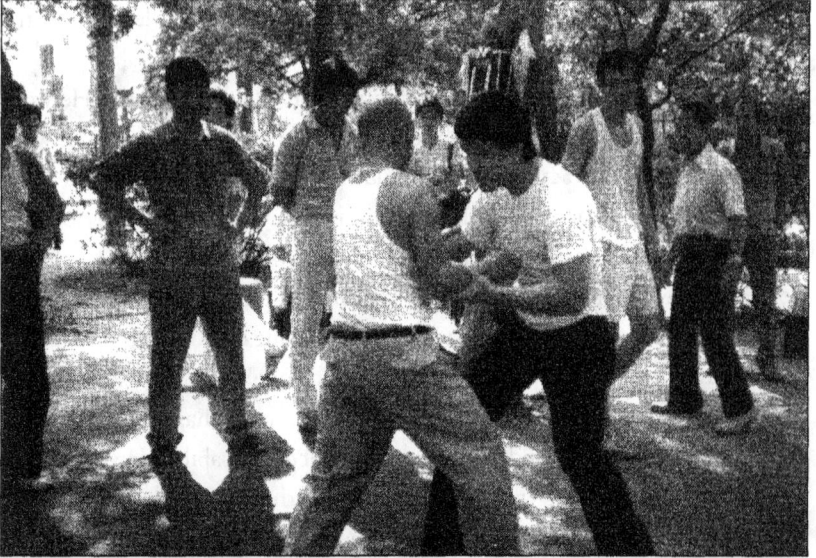

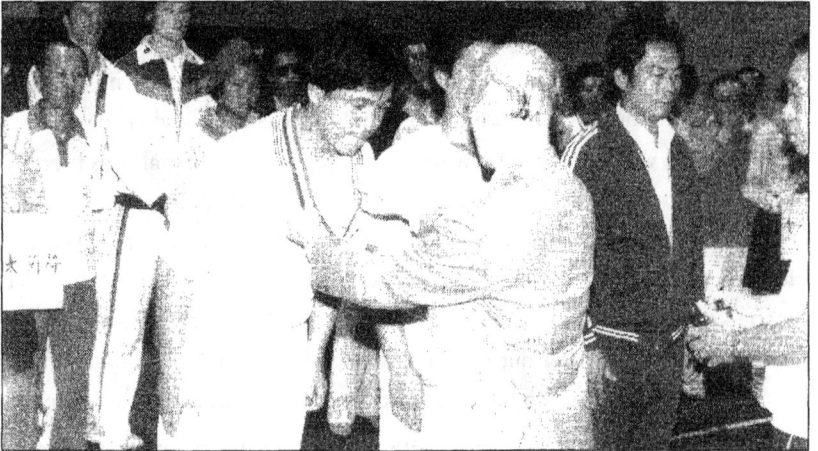

TOP: *Henry practicing push hands in Taipei's New Park, early 1980's.*
BOTTOM: *Henry receiving medal for push hands competition.*

CHAPTER FOUR

Coming to Canada

To be perfectly honest, I was not convinced that I wanted Henry or any tai chi master to come and teach in Powell River. I described earlier the obligations involved in Chinese society when one invites someone to his or her home. I realized we would be responsible for Henry in many ways. He would be living in our home, depending upon us for almost everything and complicating our very busy lives. It was really Ronnie who encouraged Henry to apply for a Canadian work visa, and she was the eternal optimist that all would turn out for the best. I, meanwhile, went along with the idea, secretly thinking it was doomed to fail.

Today I usually get all the credit for Henry's move to Canada. I tell people it was really Ronnie, but they don't want to believe me. I certainly became involved once he arrived, but Ronnie did the groundwork. This seems to be a pattern in our relationship. She gets things going and I follow through and continue the process. For Henry, the male-female issue was also a major factor. He was comfortable with me as a male, and except for tai chi we could communicate as equals. With Ronnie and other women it was more complicated. In China and Taiwan, women don't have the same status as men. Women's opinions are not highly regarded, and they are expected to defer to men. While in Taiwan, we were aware of these gender issues but did not realize they would follow us home. Thus Henry would communicate with me rather than Ronnie, who was actually doing all the work on his behalf.

Upon our return to Canada, Ronnie put her organizing skills in motion and formed the Powell River Tai Chi Association, whose purpose was to promote tai chi in the community and find a qualified teacher. She realized, of course, that there was no capable Canadian for the job and that Canadian Immigration needed to be similarly convinced in order to obtain a visa for Henry. She also approached Malaspina College, our local community college, and they agreed to hire Henry to teach tai chi classes. All was set for Henry to arrive in the fall of 1986.

Henry likes to be spontaneous and act "in the now." I'm used to this endearing trait now, but in 1986, it was a new experience. In the late spring of 1986, we received a cursory telegram from Henry, saying his arrival was imminent. This was not convenient for us at all. Students could not be expected to attend summer sessions. Furthermore I had planned a four week sailing cruise around Vancouver Island, and Ronnie was attending a workshop in California. We tried to phone Henry but misplaced his number. I can still hear the Taiwan information operator laughing when I asked her to look up Wang in the Taipei directory. We sent him a telegram asking him to delay his travel till September, as previously agreed upon. We then hoped for the best and went on our respective journeys.

Our family planned to meet in Vancouver for three days at the Expo '86 fair before returning to Powell River. Expo was fun and very crowded. On our second day we arranged to meet friends at a certain time and place. Because of the crowds, it took us half an hour to find each other despite our plans. After the relief of finally getting together, I looked out at the mass of humanity and saw Henry nonchalantly walking toward us! He had arrived in Vancouver the day before and stayed with a Chinese friend. He told her he wanted to go to Expo since he felt we might be there. We had never told him we would be in Vancouver.

We didn't have a lot of options at that point. Henry accompanied us back to our home, where he was to stay for six months. To our amazement, he was able to attract over eighty students during this period, both in Powell River and on Vancouver Island. We were to discover that Henry never worries about things working out for the best. He has absolute faith that all will be okay. He teaches that one fundamental of Daoist philosophy is called "wu wei" in Mandarin. He interprets this to mean living in the moment and being flexible with what life presents. It does not imply lack of planning, but rather a willingness to change plans if required by a new situation.

What is it like to have a tai chi master live with you for six months as part of the family? Living with Henry was never dull. First I need to explain the culture shock Henry encountered. We live in a remote area two ferry boat rides away from Vancouver, and a twenty-five minute drive from the main town of Powell River. We built our own home in a rustic manner on forty acres of land in the forest and still use an outdoor toilet. This is totally unlike Henry's life in the city of Taipei. To our pleasant surprise, he loved our home and life style. He loved the natural beauty and enjoyed walking on trails and exploring. He enjoyed meeting our friends and was interested in everything he encountered. Language was a problem for him, but he was eager to learn.

He never seemed to get lonely or bored. Ronnie and I had to go to work each day, and the kids attended school. Henry practiced tai chi for hours each day, explored the countryside, and taught classes at Malaspina College. The students loved him, and often invited him to visit them or go fishing. When we were together at home, he wanted me to be his constant companion. This caused some resentment from Ronnie and the children, and I sometimes felt caught in the middle.

He would wait for me to arrive home and then take me aside to practice tai chi. From his perspective, this was his gift to me. However, I was in conflict, because I wanted to spend time with my children or help Ronnie in meal preparation or care of the house. As a Chinese man, he felt that was Ronnie's job, and the kids could take care of themselves. I would get up from a meal to clear the table and do the dishes, and Henry would tell me to stop and let Ronnie do it while we discussed tai chi. Ronnie and I spent a lot of hours try-

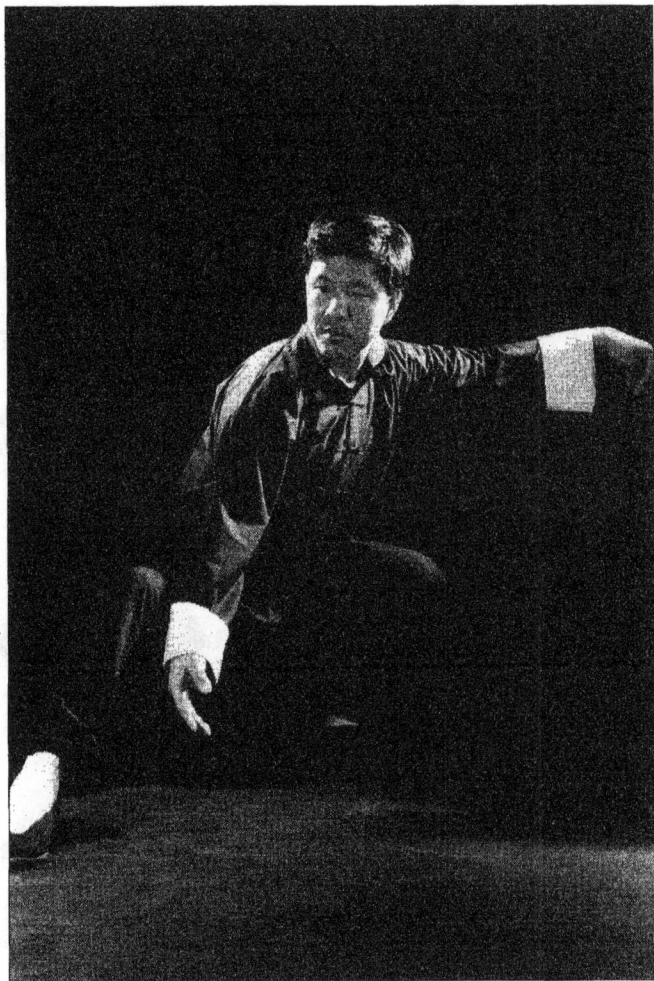

Henry practicing "Snake Creeps Down."

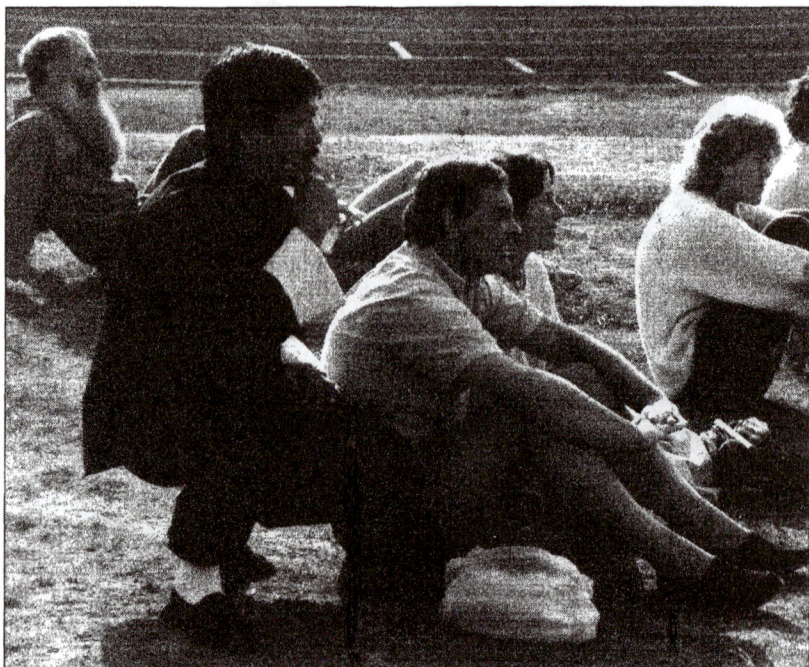

Henry's students at Malaspina College, Powell River, 1986.

ing to resolve the situation. Though I loved the opportunity to practice my Mandarin and study tai chi, the conflicting demands from family and master were quite stressful. Henry also complained that I spent too much time at work and needed to devote more time to tai chi. Since he had nothing else to do but tai chi, I resented his comments. In retrospect I realize I had not fully appreciated what it means to serve a master, and what a privilege it was to have him in our home. I was fighting against cultural differences that I didn't understand at the time. I would act differently now.

We would joke about Henry's appetite. He said that all tai chi masters have large appetites because of the energy generated as chi. Appetite was measured in numbers of bowls of rice consumed at one meal. Grandmaster Huang reputedly ate eight bowls. Sometimes I would call Henry "Chirfu" which was a pun on the word "Shirfu" or master. "Chirfu" meant a master of eating. Henry adapted quickly to western food, eating almost anything. Sometimes we would come home to find that he had prepared Chinese food for us.

I imagined what it would be like to be an art student and have Picasso living in my home. The opportunity to study and learn from a great teacher would be in conflict with my life's routine. How much do I try to stay in control? How much do I let go? One night Henry and I were doing push hands on my front porch. I suddenly felt overwhelmed with emotion and tears came to my eyes. I appreciated for the first time what a gift Henry was in my life. I was able to tell him how glad I was that he chose to live with us and how important he really was in our lives. He responded in a way that told me we were as important to him. We were becoming family to him. Moreover, we were family who finally appreciated him for what he could offer.

Looking back, I realize that Henry was incredibly adaptable and tried to understand and accept our way of doing things. So many little differences would appear. For example, students would give Henry money for classes. In Taiwan this was an insult. There his students placed their tuition fee in an envelope and left it on a desk for him. In Taiwan he was called Shirfu or Master, but Canadians would casually call him Henry. Also he expected to be thanked each time he corrected a student in class, but most students took his help for granted. Students were also unaware of the need to advise Henry if they had to miss a class. Part of my role in class was explaining his culture to the students, and the student's behaviour to him. He called me his "da tu di" or head student. This was really a great honour for me. Unfortunately, it did not imply that I was the most proficient student.

In the winter of 1986, he decided to return to Taipei. He was lonely for his family, and this was the longest he had ever been away. His tai chi courses were a great success, and he was gaining a reputation in other communities. He wanted us to continue our efforts to help him immigrate on a permanent basis. He told us that Canada would prove the proper environment for his personal tai chi growth. With a mixture of sadness and relief we took him to the airport for his flight.

PROPORTION

左右對稱

CHAPTER FIVE

Karma

As a psychiatrist, one of my favourite therapeutic tools is psychodrama. Created in 1923 by a European psychiatrist, Moreno, psychodrama provides patients the opportunity to learn about their unconscious conflicts through acting them out in a group therapy format. From the group members, a patient will choose people to play important roles in his/her life, such as parent, spouse, child, and so on. There appears to be an unconscious ability to choose the perfect group member to play the role. This "sixth sense" or intuition is called a "telerelationship" in psychodrama terminology. We all experience this phenomenon when we enter a room of strangers, and find ourselves being attracted to some people and repelled by others, despite not knowing any of them.

An example of telerelationship happened to me at a psychodrama workshop in New Zealand. I arrived on the first day unfamiliar with any of the workshop participants. The workshop leader asked the group for a volunteer to demonstrate the technique. A young woman offered to come on stage and tell her problem. She was very upset by an interaction earlier that day with her own therapist. The leader asked her to choose someone to act the role of her therapist, and after looking around the room she chose me. After a brief role play, she became visibly upset and told the leader, "He is exactly like my therapist!" She had no way of knowing I was a psychiatrist. There was no other psychiatrist in the group.

Later when I studied with Dr. Elizabeth Kubler-Ross, she described how we come across people in our lives who force us to look at ourselves. These people

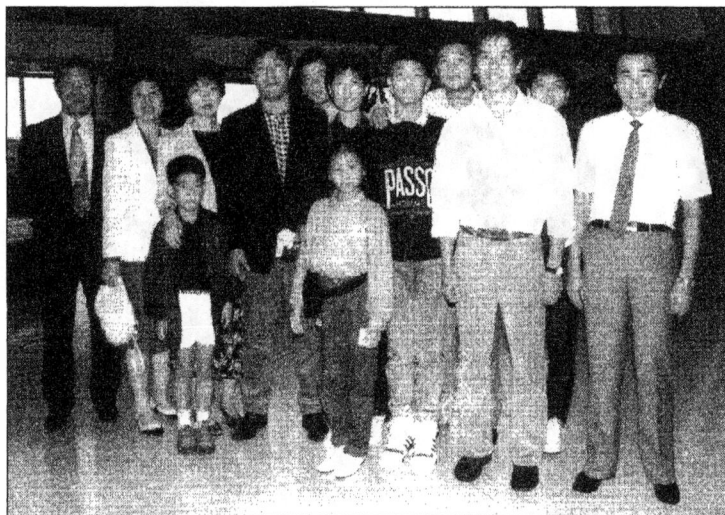

Henry and family leaving Taiwan for Canada, October 1987

may trigger emotions we don't fully understand, such as anger, fear, jealousy, grief, love, etc. She calls these people "gifts" to emphasize the benefits their interactions provide. Most of us have difficulty appreciating these "gifts," but they do offer the prospect of growth and change in our lives.

Henry is an incredible "gift" in my life. Even when we are physically distant, he influences my life. I am never fully comfortable or relaxed around him, and he constantly pushes against my personal boundaries. I am forced to look at myself, my lifestyle, values, and goals. He acts as a mirror for me to reflect upon.

Once when Henry was living at our house, he saw a large dead fir tree in our front yard. He told me I should cut it down, and I replied that I planned to hire someone to do the job. I told him I did not feel confident to cut the tree down myself. I was also afraid. He said he would help me though he had never even seen a tree being felled. Despite my objections he convinced me to get my chainsaw and start cutting. He would periodically look at the saw cut

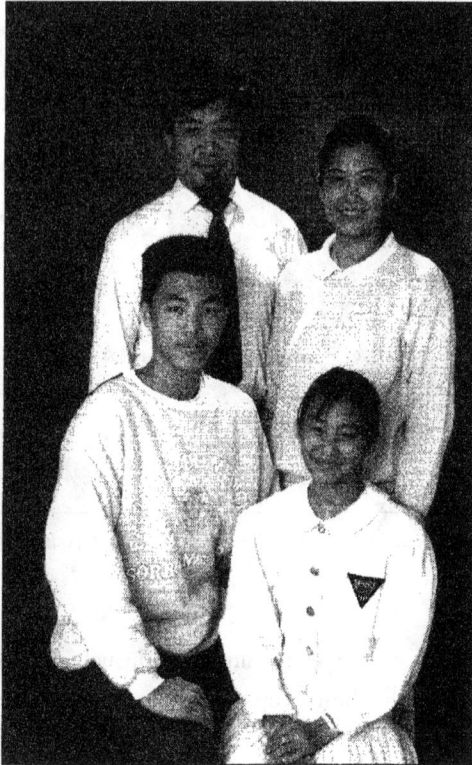

Henry, Ivy, David, and Amy after arrival in Canada.

and the tree, and tell me what to do next. The end result was a tree which fell exactly where it was meant to go. I also felt more confidence in my own abilities, which Henry never questioned.

We also have a strong telerelationship, or unconscious connection. He uses the term "karma" to describe our relationship. I think he means that fate has brought us together, and fate will determine our future together. A friend of mine who leads workshops in past life regression felt that Henry and I shared previous lifetimes together, and in one of these past lives we were native Indians and brothers. Certainly Henry and I are closely bonded in this lifetime.

Henry's first trip to Canada had triggered some personal issues for me. One choice I had made in life was to be an active, involved husband and parent. This was clearly a reaction to my own parents, who chose their careers as a priority. In particular, my father, a world-renowned cancer specialist, worked long hours, travelled frequently, and published extensively. When he was home, our interaction was on his terms, and he showed little interest in my life. I'm sure my choice to enter medicine was partly influenced by my desire to share more with my father. Even this failed as he preferred to talk about his medical career, rather than mine.

Henry's single-mindedness about tai chi reminds me of my father's dedication to cancer treatment. Henry puts his study and teaching of tai chi before everything else in his life. Certainly his family has had to accommodate his life choices. Since he is clear about his path in life, he expects his students to make similar choices. He feels if we are serious about learning tai chi, it should be our priority. He has told me several times that each person is meant to focus on one thing in life, and for him that is obviously tai chi.

So far I have not been able to make such a clear choice in my life. As a result my tai chi skills have not reached a level that satisfies me. My sense is that very few of us can commit our lives to a single purpose, and only those who do can become masters. How much time and effort I devote to tai chi is an ongoing issue for me. While Henry lived in our home, I faced this issue daily. After he returned to Taiwan, his absence allowed me time to process all that transpired during his visit.

We kept contact with Henry while he and his family contemplated moving permanently to Powell River. For a Taiwanese family to move to a remote community with no familiar ties was not an easy decision.

Interested tai chi students from Powell River and Vancouver Island communities as far away as Victoria, who had studied with Henry, offered to assist with his immigration application. Many wrote letters of support and indicated to the Canadian authorities they would attend tai chi classes, allowing Henry to be self-supporting. One student even had "guanxi" with an immigration official in Hong Kong, who was processing the Wang family's applications. Was this another example of Henry's faith that everything will work out for the best?

On October 24, 1987, I met the Wangs at Vancouver International Airport and drove them to Powell River. Just prior to their arrival a patient of mine told me she had to attend a therapy program in Vancouver for two months. She was unable to find someone to sublet her home and feared she couldn't afford to attend the program. Of course the timing was perfect and the Wangs moved into a beautiful furnished home until more permanent placement could be found.

Henry also decided he needed a vehicle, and the first local car dealer we approached suggested a used station wagon that had just arrived. We phoned our own mechanic for advice. He told us that the car belonged to his best friend and that he had performed all the servicing himself. He actually advised us to buy the car for our own use! So in a community with limited house rentals and few used car options, Henry found a lovely home and an excellent automobile. Two months later our Taiwanese friend, Diana, offered the Wangs a large house to rent. She also became close friends with Henry and his family, and helped them cope with a new and different lifestyle.

The Wang family quickly adjusted to Powell River life. Ronnie and I brainstormed, and suggested several English names for their two children. They chose David and Amy. It's not often we get to name someone else's children! Ivy took on the responsibilities of daily living, and the kids attended local schools. The kids quickly made Canadian friends and started to learn English. David especially enjoyed fishing in a nearby lake. Henry soon had several classes of tai chi students. He also arranged tai chi workshops around the province and in Europe. I accompanied Henry to as many classes and workshops as my own schedule would allow. We also met on a personal basis to socialize and practice tai chi.

CHAPTER SIX

Daily Practice

On an early spring morning, I am out in my front yard practicing tai chi. It's six thirty, and the sun is not yet visible through the fir trees surrounding my house. There is a chill in the air which keeps the early morning insects away. In another few weeks, I'll be forced to practice on my front porch which is screened to keep out the annoying little critters. It is customary to practice tai chi early in the morning. Henry usually starts around five thirty, even in the winter. I try to discipline myself to get up at six thirty. Okay, sometimes it's seven or later. I do practice every day. Almost. In China, most people get up very early, even in the dark, and go outside to a park to practice. My cynical nature believes that the Chinese practice tai chi as a way of providing a haven of personal space in a crowded society of one billion people.

Ancient Chinese lore states that the world's energy changes every two hours in a cyclical fashion. Therefore morning and evening are considered optimal times to practice tai chi. Of course one can practice at any time. One positive aspect of early morning practice is less distraction. The phone hasn't started to ring, the rest of the family is sleeping, and work is still a couple of hours away. I don't play any music since I want to focus inward and be sensitive only to the natural sounds around me. It's a wonderful way to start my day and gets me relaxed and centred. On those days that I don't practice, or rush through my form, my body can feel the difference. Just as my body lets me know when I am hungry or tired, it also tells me when I need to play my tai chi.

Tai chi is very portable, requiring only a small practice area. I have practiced at home, on the beach, on mountain tops, at ferry landings, hotel

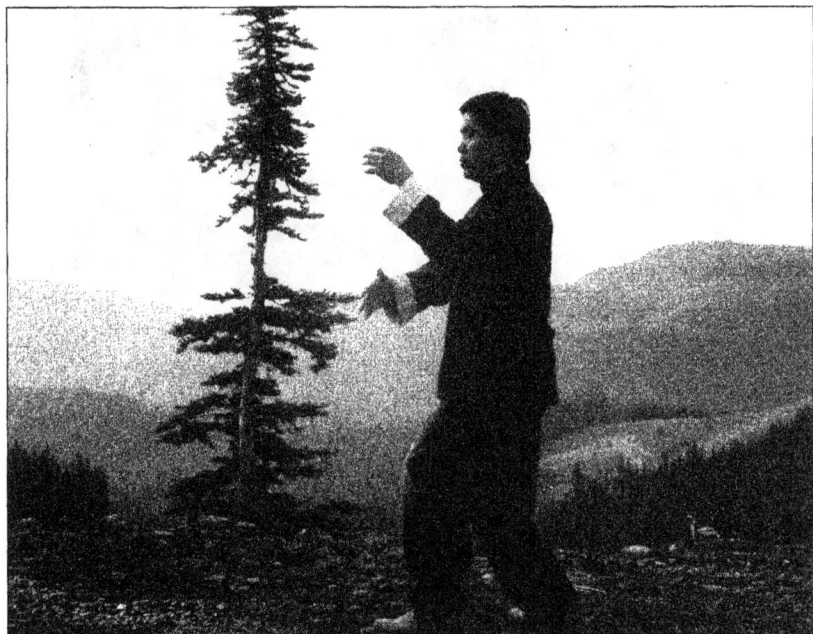

Henry practicing Tai Chi form.

rooftops, and ashrams in India, to name only a few locations. Each place provides unique energy which I try to absorb into my body while practicing my form. The surrounding energy will depend on the time of day, the climatic conditions, and natural environs.

Henry stresses the importance of regular daily practice. He practices four hours every day, sometimes more, depending on his teaching schedule. Practice should not be meaningless repetition of tai chi postures. When I practice, I try to apply what was learned in a recent lesson. I also try to determine where my form needs improvement or where my energy seems blocked. Then I can take questions to Henry at my next class.

This morning, and most mornings, I start my routine with some warm up exercises to get my body relaxed and ready for the tai chi form. These exercises involve bending the spine, turning the waist and relaxing the shoulders.

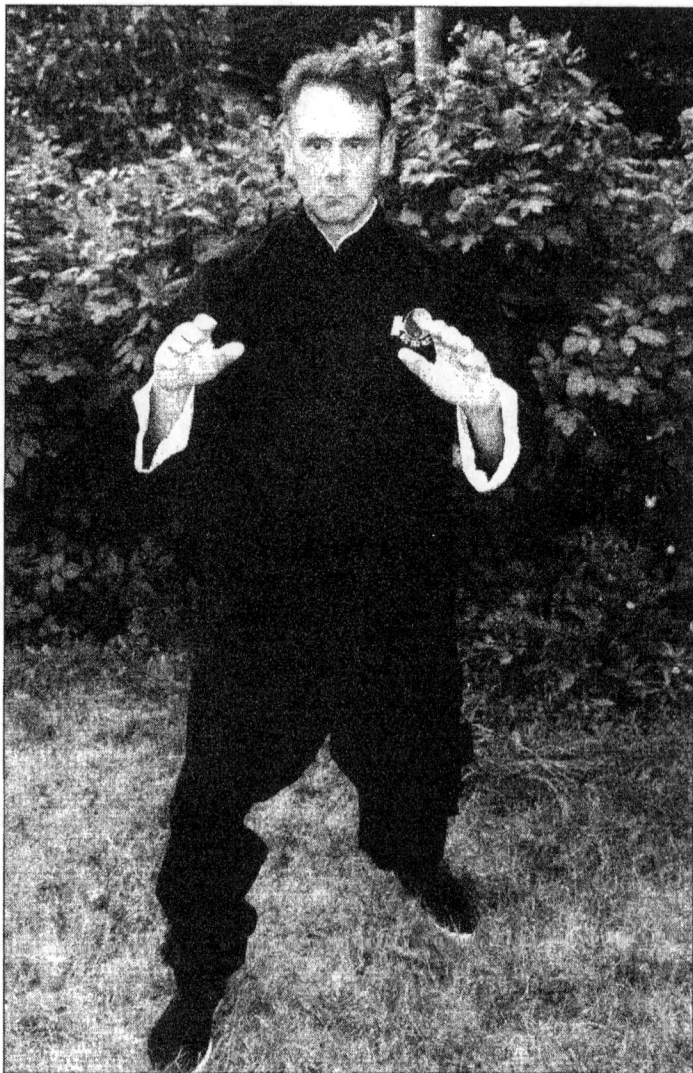

Author in Powell River practicing Tai Chi form.

I am always gentle with my body and avoid pushing beyond comfortable limits. Tai chi is not about "no pain – no gain." Often I can hear or feel my joints loosening and popping as I get softer. Sometimes I add some stretch exercises as well, which mostly involve my legs and back. These beginning exercises are similar to "qi gong" which is gaining in popularity. Tai chi and qi gong are really based on the same concept. The difference is that qi gong emphasizes single postures, rather than a sequential form, and also focuses more on breathing patterns.

I am now ready to practice my form. The Chinese use the term "playing" tai chi, which I feel is appropriate. When I first learned tai chi in Vancouver, I studied a long form composed of one hundred and eight positions. It took me almost a year to learn it all. My main focus at that time was just remembering the total sequence and keeping my concentration. Any time my mind was distracted, I would lose my place. Though I was not aware at the time, I was learning tai chi as traditionally taught. This means that I followed my master's moves and tried to copy him. There were aspects of this form that I would later have to unlearn and change under Henry's instruction. I will discuss the differences between traditional tai chi and Henry's concepts later.

In my daily practice I start with section one of the Cheng Man-Ching modified Yang style. This form comprises thirty seven movements divided into three sections for easier study. In reality there are more than thirty seven movements since several movements are repeated. Also, as one of Henry's students, I learned to practice the form from both the right and left sides. This allows for balance and symmetry. Traditional teachers instruct students to learn only one side.

I will usually repeat section one several times, then move on to sections two and three. These latter sections have some kicks which demand more timing and balance than section one. While playing at my form, my mind is constantly assessing each movement. Henry teaches us to consider seven basic tai chi principles while practicing. These consist of centre, balance, relaxation, concentration, circle, coordination, and proportion. I will discuss these in detail later.

The tai chi form requires constant practice to do correctly. The essence of tai chi is in any single tai chi posture. Henry calls this "one form." It is not really necessary to study hundreds of movements or styles. Many students of tai chi feel that more is better and learn several styles. They also study use of weapons, such as swords, poles, and knives. Personally, I would be extremely happy to feel competent in the short form I study. I have no desire to dilute my skills by learning more movements. The seven principles which apply to all styles of tai chi are of basic importance.

It takes me approximately one hour to complete my morning practice. After finishing the third section for the final time, I will remain quietly in the closing posture for a couple of minutes to feel the chi circulate in my body. Hopefully there will be some evidence of chi flow, such as a feeling of warmth inside. Sometimes I experience tingling sensations in my hands or moisture on my palms. Since tai chi is not an aerobic workout, my pulse and breathing should be normal or slowed in rate.

Finally I rub my palms together in a circular manner and then massage my face, ears, knees, and back using circular movements. This is supposed to transmit chi energy to those parts of the body and promote healing. In particular, massaging the ears will stimulate several important acupuncture points. My dog has learned that this massage heralds the end to my tai chi exercises, so he usually starts whining for me to take him on a walk.

Tai chi concepts should be practiced all day. When my dog and I take our walk, I continue to focus on the seven principles, especially relaxation. Driving is another time when I need to remember to relax my neck and shoulders. Henry teaches us to move our bodies correctly when doing activities such as chopping wood, shoveling in the garden, hiking, rowing, etc. In this fashion tai chi becomes more and more a part of life, and not just an isolated morning routine.

I attend Henry's class once a week. In addition to participating in his advanced class, I also assist at his intermediate and beginning classes. During class he will answer student questions and clarify any confusion. From our

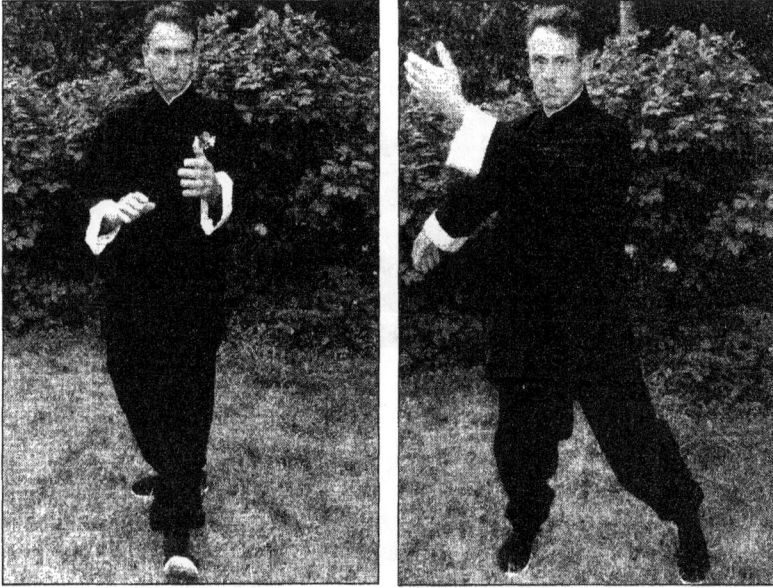

Author in Powell River practicing Tai Chi form.

questions he knows who has been practicing. We will review one or two sections of the form together and then focus on one or two moves in particular. If
there is time, he will ask us to practice "search centre," which is his personal
concept of push hands. Search centre is an application of the tai chi form, and
is generally taught to students who have completed study of the form. It is
performed with a partner, and the players develop sensitivity to each other's
energy. Search centre and tai chi form are interrelated and connected by the
seven principles. A detailed explanation of search centre will follow later.

Though I try to follow a regular daily tai chi routine, each day's experience
is unique. My performance of the form is never the same, and I am always
learning something new. Henry once told me that daily practice is similar to
regular deposits of money into a bank account.

BALANCE

重心穩固

CHAPTER SEVEN

Chinese Culture

Tai chi is Chinese. This simple truism has great implications. To appreciate tai chi I also have to understand some of the differences between Chinese culture and my own. I have travelled to Taiwan twice and China four times. I have visited these countries as a tourist and also as a visiting professor of psychiatry. Over the years I have studied the language, history, and philosophy of China. I love Chinese cuisine. Yet I still feel an outsider. Indeed that is what the Chinese call us: "wai guo ren" or "outside the country person." Even in Canada, a Chinese person will refer to a non-Chinese Canadian citizen as an "outsider."

In describing my relationship with Henry, I have already alluded to some of our cultural differences. Sometimes there have been misunderstandings and always an attempt to find a common ground. Some differences seem minor but are worth addressing. Learning to say "Shirfu" or Master is an important sign of respect. Saying thank you is considered more than a polite formality. Putting money in an envelope prior to paying for lessons is easy to do. Acknowledging the master-student relationship is a major component of tai chi.

For me a major difficulty is balancing my relationship with my master with the rest of my life. Henry has always generously offered himself to me, my family, and his students. From the Chinese perspective the master-student bond is intimate and forever. It is not to be taken lightly. Most of Henry's students, myself included, do not really appreciate this. I still do not avail myself of Henry's generosity. I could study with him any time I wished, and yet I don't take advantage of this often enough. I convince myself that I have more important things to do. I still don't really "get it."

Henry is generous in many ways. He often invites me to stay with his family and share in his life. He moved from Powell River to Comox, British Columbia, on Vancouver Island. In Comox there is a larger population base from which to draw students. Also there is easier access to the other communities where he teaches. In addition, the Island provides a cleaner environment compared to Powell River, with its large paper mill. Nevertheless he has continued to take a ferry once a week to teach his Powell River classes. I feel this is an example of his personal commitment to Ronnie and me, as well as his dedication to his pupils.

Due to the move, we see less of each other. We keep in regular contact, and I enjoy visiting Henry. Ivy's cooking alone is worth the trip. There is also lots of time for tai chi practice. On Sunday mornings students meet in a school yard near Henry's home for free practice sessions. I join them when possible.

I don't think that Henry's teachers were so giving. He states that his schooling was more traditional. He mentions how his teachers would not explain things in the detail that he does with us. He laughingly describes how masters would wear long gowns that covered their legs and hid the "secrets" of their movements. They might only demonstrate a move to him once and expect him to understand it. He had to struggle to learn tai chi while he offers it to us on a platter. I know he has difficulty understanding our seeming lack of appreciation. It appears that we take his teaching for granted.

The tai chi master-student relationship issue has arisen often. Once Henry, my friend Steve, and I went for a hike in the mountains outside Comox. Henry was teaching me how to walk using tai chi principles. He asked me to pick up a rock from the path and walk with it in one hand to study the effects of the rock on my balance and centre. After stopping for a snack break we continued on our way. Ten minutes passed when Henry noticed I no longer was carrying the rock. I told him that I left the rock where we had stopped to eat. He was obviously upset and told me to backtrack and retrieve the same rock. I realized the rock was irrelevant, but obeying my master was the real issue. I returned to fetch the rock.

One year during a summer workshop at Mt. Washington, in British Columbia, he finished teaching some aspect of the solo tai chi form and told his students to move to a different place to study "search centre," his version of tai chi pushing hands practice. Some students lagged behind to continue practicing the form concepts they had just studied. He told the students who followed him that the others had not obeyed him and implied it would be difficult for them to learn tai chi properly.

Once an accomplished tai chi player visited Henry. He was unwilling to acknowledge Henry as his master yet wanted to learn his search centre concepts. Henry was very polite but refused to practice with the man. Instead Henry let him practice with some senior students, and the man left for home quite angry and hurt. Later Henry said that the tai chi player's "glass is full of water. I can't add any more."

Some of my non tai chi friends wonder why I humble myself before my master, and comply with his requests. I realize that in our tai chi relationship he is my master, and for me to learn from him requires letting go of my ego. Letting go is the basic teaching of tai chi. In martial arts if a student is unwilling to lose, they will never learn how to win. This is also called "investment in loss."

Henry also has had to "let go" of many customs since moving to Canada. He has had to adapt to our western practices much more than we have accepted his. He has tried to retain the most valuable Chinese customs and incorporate them in his life in Canada.

Henry has a metaphor which describes letting go and investing in loss. He asks his students to imagine a large jagged boulder entering the top of a mountain stream. As the rock travels down the mountain, it gets tossed and bounced against the stream bed and eroded by air and water. By the time it reaches the base of the mountain its rough edges have been worn away, and its shape is round. As a round boulder it is less vulnerable to further damage.

In tai chi push hands practice, two opponents spar with each other, trying to knock the other person off balance. As long as one stays "hard" and resists being pushed, their opponent can easily find their centre of balance and win. On the other hand, if one stays "soft" and lets go, one's centre will be more difficult to contact. To develop this softness requires a willingness to lose for a time. Many students are unwilling to lose in the short term, not really believing that lack of resistance will triumph in the long term.

As my life continues, I realize more and more the value of letting go and not resisting. In my work as a psychiatrist there are many times I have tried to encourage patients to do things my way. Often they concur, and there is no problem. When they resist me, it is tempting to keep on imposing my position. Tai chi has taught me that it is better in most instances to simply state my opinion and then let the patients choose their own path based on all the information provided. Most times this has proven to be the best course for all concerned. Rather than try to walk through a wall, I opt for opening the door.

This path of least resistance is not to be confused with giving up or losing. The Chinese use the example of grass bending in a strong wind and surviving, while a stiff tree will break and be destroyed. Similarly when trying to land a fish, I will let the line slack when the fish runs, and reel in when it's tired. When trying to move a cow it is easier to offer it hay than try pushing or pulling. Tai chi philosophy teaches that soft will overcome hard and "four ounces can move a thousand pounds."

COORDINATION

移動全動

CHAPTER EIGHT

Learning to Let Go

Most famous tai chi masters are also proficient at several traditional Chinese arts, such as calligraphy, painting, poetry, acupuncture, and herbal medicine. Grandmaster Cheng Man-Ching has been called "the master of five excellences." Henry has also devoted much of his life to studying Chinese medicine, calligraphy, and Daoist philosophy. Everywhere he travels, he carries with him some Chinese herbal remedies and acupuncture needles. If a student in class has any somatic complaints, Henry will usually recommend some dietary change, some herbal medicine, and acupuncture needles. He treated my daughter Tai's painful wrist with two needles and cured her symptoms in one treatment.

Since moving to Comox, Henry has attempted to master two other less traditional disciplines: real estate and gardening. At one point I counted more real estate agents at Henry's home than tai chi students. Actually some agents did join his classes. Part of his interest in real estate was trying to find a place that would entice me away from Powell River. He would pick me up from the ferry landing and instead of driving me back to his home, he would take us to some property he was convinced I would love. He wanted so much for my family to move close to him.

He had much more luck with his family and friends back in Taiwan. Probably fuelled by fears of Taiwan's future takeover by Mainland China, many Taiwanese were investing in Canada. He arranged for some close family and friends to buy properties in the Comox valley, and these have only risen in value. He also convinced his parents to buy a home in Vancouver. They come

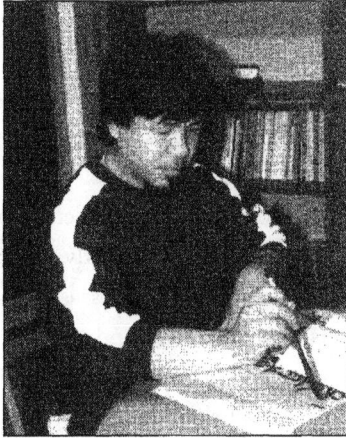

Henry practicing calligraphy.

once or twice a year for a brief visit but usually avoid visiting Comox. They do not speak English and find Comox too isolated, small, and boring. They love Vancouver where Chinese is spoken everywhere.

Henry has also been searching for a tai chi "home." He envisions a place where he and his family can live, and where students will come from near and far to study tai chi and related arts. He wants a place that will be convenient for students to reach, but also one of natural beauty and tranquility. We have looked at many prospective properties together, but none has yet been suitable. Our tai chi centre is still a dream but hopefully an eventual reality.

When we weren't looking at real estate, we were going to nurseries and garden shops. Henry and Ivy both love to garden and are quite knowledgeable. Henry was not too proficient at conversational English, but quickly learned the names of all the plants in the area. Though Ronnie shared their enthusiasm of all things green and growing, I found gardening of minimal interest.

Once Henry and I went to a nearby nursery. He found a fir tree on sale for twenty five dollars and went to the counter to pay. The salesperson charged him thirty dollars. When we asked about the price difference, he showed us a tag on the tree which clearly stated thirty dollars. After carrying the tree home to Henry's, we noticed that the tree carried two tags. One said thirty dollars, while the other said twenty five dollars. I told Henry that he should only have had to pay the lower price. We drove back to the nursery, and Henry asked me to explain the situation, since I spoke English.

The salesperson listened to me, and then called for his wife to make a decision. She listened to my explanation impatiently. Then quite rudely she told me that the lower price was from the previous season and that we were getting a bargain at thirty dollars. I was surprised and upset by her comments. I also felt I had failed in getting justice for Henry. I told him in Mandarin what was being said, and asked him what I should do. He told me to forget about the money and return to his home.

On the drive home, Henry explained to me that it was not worth arguing over five dollars. Also he said if I were to fight with the owner, she would just feel more justified in her position. By our "letting go" she perhaps will wonder if she did the correct thing or if she lost a future customer. This was another lesson for me in non-resistance.

I learned a similar lesson in a totally different situation. A karate teacher in Powell River approached me, and asked if she could observe one of Henry's tai chi classes. I was quite excited since I was sure she would be very impressed by Henry's martial art skills. Henry agreed that she could sit on the side of the classroom and observe. That class consisted of some tai chi form instruction and later search centre practice. Watching the class would have been about as interesting as watching paint dry

I mentioned to Henry that the karate teacher was probably bored, and that it might be more interesting for her if she could practice search centre with him directly. He told me that if she was interested in tai chi, she should sign up for lessons with him. He was obviously uninterested in proving anything to anyone. I realized that I was trying to use Henry to impress the karate teacher. It was my ego involved, not Henry's!

CHAPTER NINE

The Seven Principles

One of Henry's teaching tools is the video camera. He is regularly video-taping his tai chi form and search centre techniques. He then studies the tapes and corrects any faults in his practice. He also films students so that they can see what they need to work on. I am unable to really see myself when I am doing my tai chi form, so watching myself on video is extremely valuable. I can always find areas in my body that are stiff or tense, and where Henry's seven principles have not been followed. Video is also valuable in search centre practice, where slow motion can be utilized to reveal actions that are too quick to observe naturally.

Recently Henry invited me to view a tape he made in 1986 while he was teaching students at Malaspina College in Powell River. I was unprepared for what I saw. Henry was demonstrating the form, but his form has changed dramatically in the past ten years. Being with Henry on a day-to-day basis has caused me to miss the bigger picture. Also my own ability has improved to the point where I can now recognize details that I was previously unaware of. Since coming to Canada, Henry has been able to carefully study tai chi and formulate new concepts. His application of these ideas is evident in the way his tai chi is performed now.

Over the years students have asked Henry to make a video they could purchase for study purposes. He has always refused, saying that he didn't want his tai chi to be "fixed" on a film. When I saw how much his tai chi has progressed through the years, I understood his reasoning. Many tai chi masters seem to reach a plateau in their tai chi process and then teach the same content to their students. Often they teach exactly what they studied from their own master, and there is no progress or fresh thought. Because of tradition they are reluctant to challenge the ideas of the famous masters.

There is much that is rich in tai chi tradition, but there is also potential to stifle new and creative ideas. Henry has developed many new possibilities for improving tai chi, but there is a general reluctance to accept them among traditional tai chi players. Sometimes I feel he is trying to convince people that the Earth is round, when they know otherwise. Henry talks about progress in other sports. For example high jumpers used a "scissors kick" for years. Then someone decided to try diving forward over the bar. More recently competitors have been winning by flipping backwards over the bar.

Grandmaster Cheng Man-Ching is a classic example of expertise in tai chi forms and pushing hands. He is revered almost like a god among tai chi players, especially in Taiwan. When I look at videos of Grandmaster Cheng, I see how Henry has departed from tradition. The Grandmaster is very soft and relaxed, and definitely has martial skills, but his pushing hands and solo form are not integrated. When pushing hands, he uses a lot of muscular force and body movement compared to Grandmaster Huang or Henry. This is not meant to criticize Grandmaster Cheng, but only to describe the evolution in tai chi that has transpired.

Henry's seven principles are the basis of his tai chi philosophy. He calls them the foundation of the house. Though he teaches the modified Yang style, he believes all other tai chi styles, and even other martial arts, should observe the same fundamentals to be effective. When I practice my tai chi form each morning, I am not just going through the paces of a mindless dance. I am attempting to move my body according to the seven principles. Often I will focus on one or two principles rather than confuse myself with all seven. Each principle is of equal importance, and they are interdependent. All must be applied properly to produce the correct results.

As I explain the seven principles, the reader must imagine that I am practicing my tai chi form. I am connecting thirty seven different movements in a fluid sequence. Each posture has evolved from ancient times and once served a martial function. I am attempting to absorb chi energy from my surroundings and circulate this chi through my body, finally transmitting energy back out into the environment, using my body and mind.

I will discuss the CENTRE principle first. Henry describes the centre of a person as their head connected through their spine and dan tien to their feet. The dan tien is located slightly below the navel and inside the abdomen, as opposed to the waist, which is on the outside of the body. The dan tien is centrally located anatomically and stores the body's chi energy. All tai chi movements must arise from the centre. Perhaps some metaphors will help to explain this concept.

The cutting power of a pair of scissors decreases the further from its central axis. Or imagine a machine with many interlocking gears. The central gear controls the movements of the outlying ones. This is an analogy for the body's centre controlling the arms and legs. When a fish swims, it uses its centre to initiate movement, not its head or tail.

I like to imagine a brace and bit used for drilling into a piece of wood. The top of the brace is similar to my head, the handle is my waist, while the bit is analogous to my feet. The tool must be centred while the handle turns for the bit to bite into the wood. If the brace is tilted off centre, it will not screw straight into the wood. In a similar fashion, the ability to centre oneself will develop the ability to "root" into the ground. I have seen Henry adopt a stance and then ask eight students to try to push him away from his position. Because he is centred, his feet seem to grow roots into the ground beneath him, and the students are unable to shift him. Following the centre principle means that I initiate my movements from my centre—my waist and trunk—then allow my extremities to follow. Henry describes how a gardener fertilizes a plant's roots and not its leaves. Move from your centre, not your arms; allowing your arms to follow.

Related to centre is weight distribution. Traditional tai chi masters teach that one's weight should be seventy percent on one foot, and thirty percent on

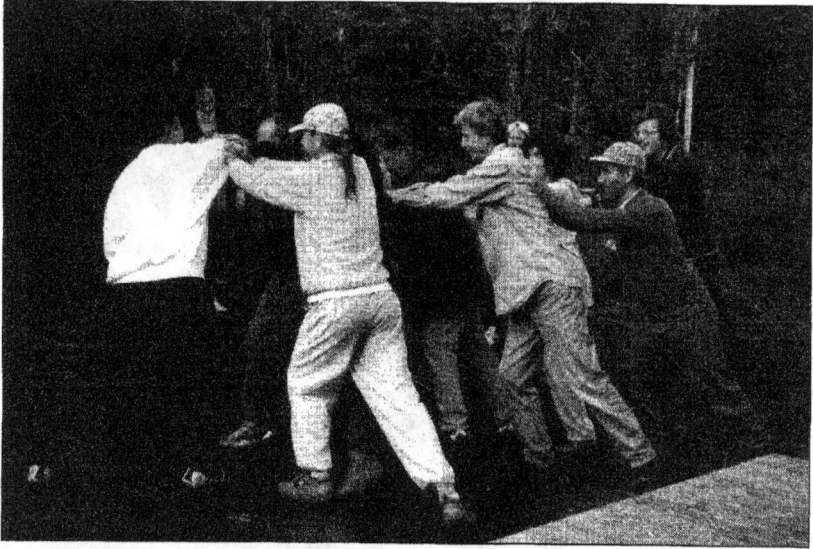

Henry "rooted" against eight students.

the other. Henry disagrees. He feels this concept places one off centre in a leaning posture. He claims this causes "double weighting," where the arm and leg on one side of the body are load bearing at the same time. This position is unnatural and can cause physical harm to the body. Furthermore, chi flow is disrupted by a seventy-thirty weight distribution.

Henry teaches us that our weight should either be one hundred percent on one foot and zero on the other, or fifty percent on each foot. Tai chi should be as natural as possible. When we stand, we naturally choose a fifty-fifty weight distribution. When we walk, we shift from a hundred-zero position to the next hundred-zero position. In class Henry attempts a demonstration of someone trying to walk using the seventy-thirty concept. Invariably this provides much amusement among the onlookers.

The philosophy of yin yang also implies harmony and equality. The tai chi symbol depicts a fifty-fifty balance of yin and yang.

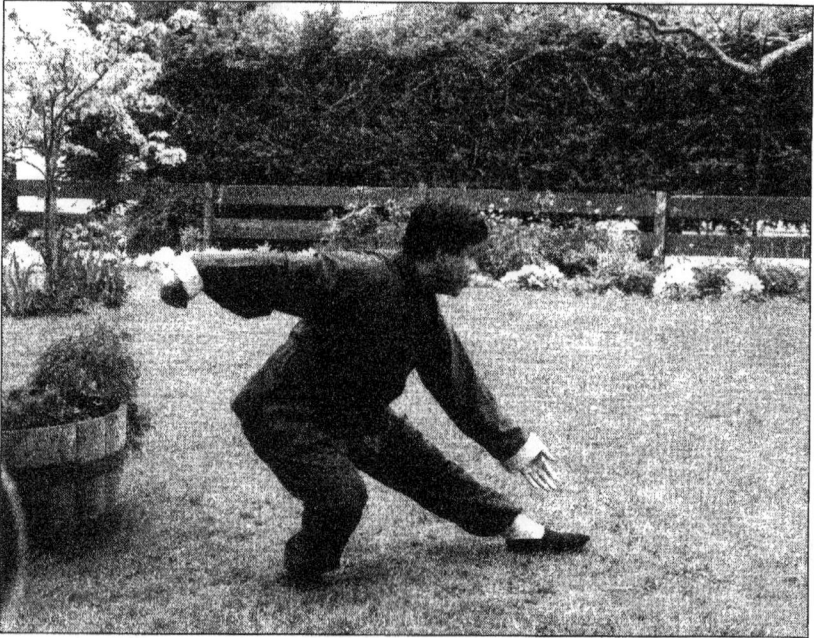

Henry demonstrating tai chi posture "Snake Creeps Down."

In my form practice I concentrate on turning my body's centre before shifting my weight from fifty-fifty to a hundred-zero or vice versa. As my weight shifts, it is really my centre which moves while my extremities follow. Also I never allow my body to move forward more than fifty-fifty. All this makes my form look quite different from that practiced by traditional players. Compared to them, I do not lean forward or backward. My front knee is never farther forward than my toes. All of my movements seem confined to a smaller radius. My arms and legs follow my body's centre, and therefore do not seem to stretch, push, or pull. I turn first and shift my weight after. My head stays connected to my spine and doesn't move independently. All the movements appear to arise from inside my body rather than outside, and energy is transmitted in a centrifugal direction.

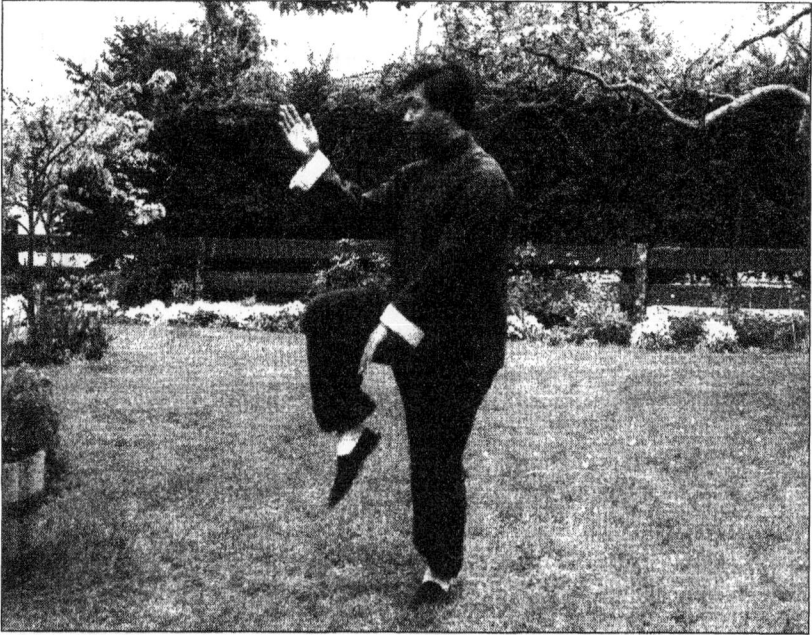

Henry demonstrating tai chi posture the "Golden Pheasant Stands on one leg."

BALANCE is the second principle. I attempt to be centred and balanced. An ice skater may demonstrate superb balancing skills yet lack centre. This is most evident when they lean while skating. With the seventy-thirty concept, there can also be balance without centre. Skiers, on the other hand, tend to utilize both principles and often use a fifty-fifty or hundred-zero weight distribution.

Balance permits fluid movement from one position to the next in a relaxed fashion. Though every posture in the solo form requires balance, there are certain positions requiring balance on one leg, or turning while standing on one leg. There are points in the separate postures where balance is most easily achieved. These natural balance points provide a foundation for the centre to turn and shift more easily.

Changing from one position to another may involve a change in direction of forty five degrees or multiples thereof, such as ninety, or one hundred and thirty five degrees. Every movement in the solo form follows this general pattern. These angles provide a stable platform for changing to the next position and therefore contribute to balance. Of course, this is difficult for someone unfamiliar with the tai chi form to comprehend.

Try to picture me facing north (0 degrees) with my left foot forward, my right foot in back. Each foot carries fifty percent of my weight. I then turn my trunk forty five degrees to the right and then shift one hundred percent of my weight to the front foot. I balance myself on that front foot, then lift up my back foot and place it forward and to the right facing east (90 degrees). Then I turn my trunk to face east and shift my centre forward to a fifty-fifty weight distribution. In a similar fashion I can continue through the form keeping balanced and centred.

When turning my centre and shifting my weight, I must also keep my body level and avoid moving up and down. In other schools of tai chi, players will often move up and down as they turn. Henry feels this contributes to tension in the hip joints and decreased ability to root oneself to the ground.

PROPORTION is the third principle. Simply stated, proportion means that my left hand is related to my right foot, my left elbow is related to my right knee, and my left shoulder is related to my right hip and vice-versa. When moving through the tai chi form I try to feel an internal connection between my arm on one side and my opposite leg. If my left knee is bent, then my right elbow must be bent proportionally. Proportion implies not only a right to left balance, but also a vertical to horizontal, and forward to backward balance.

When I am following the proportion principle, my body takes on a circular or globe shape. Someone could use a compass and draw a circle around my body, using my hands and feet as the outer circumference and my dan tien as centre. I feel as if I am inside a large ball. Any outside force touching my hands would be transmitted through my centre to my feet. Sometimes in class I will check for proportion by having another student apply force against one of my

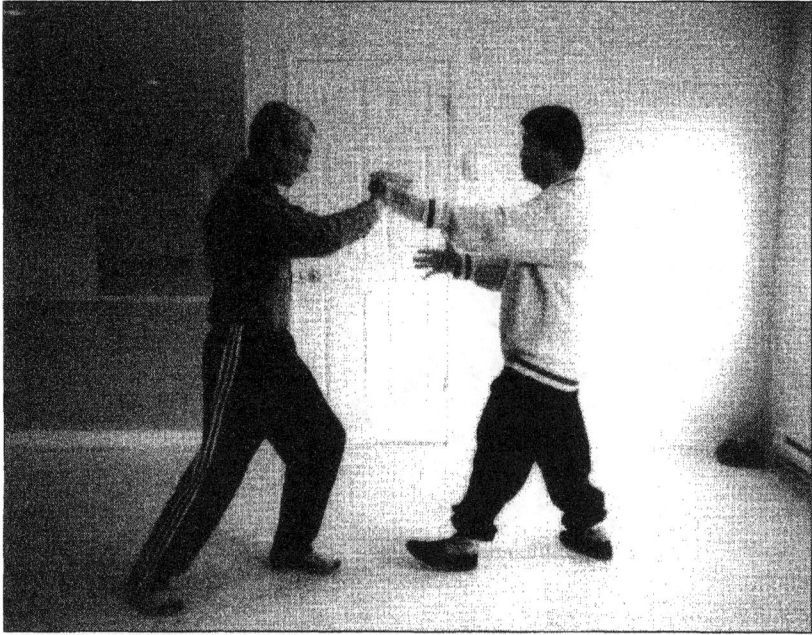

Student "testing" Master Wang's posture for connection to ground.

arms. If my stance is correct, they will feel as if they are pushing against the leg on the opposite side of the arm they are pushing. They will feel that my body is connected and rooted to the ground. Any internal chi energy would originate from my centre and radiate outwardly through my arms and legs.

The fourth principle, CIRCLE, is paramount in tai chi. I just described how I try to achieve a globe shape while my body's centre is the axis. In tai chi all movements are circular and straight lines are absent. Arms and legs are always supple and slightly curved, and their movements follow circular arcs. This insistence on circular motions is generally different from hard style martial arts. Punches in karate, for example, are often delivered in a straight line with great force. If the start of the punch contains 100% energy, then the completion of the punch is 0%, or empty. In contrast, a "punch" in tai chi is circular and the 100% energy is maintained throughout at any point on the circle.

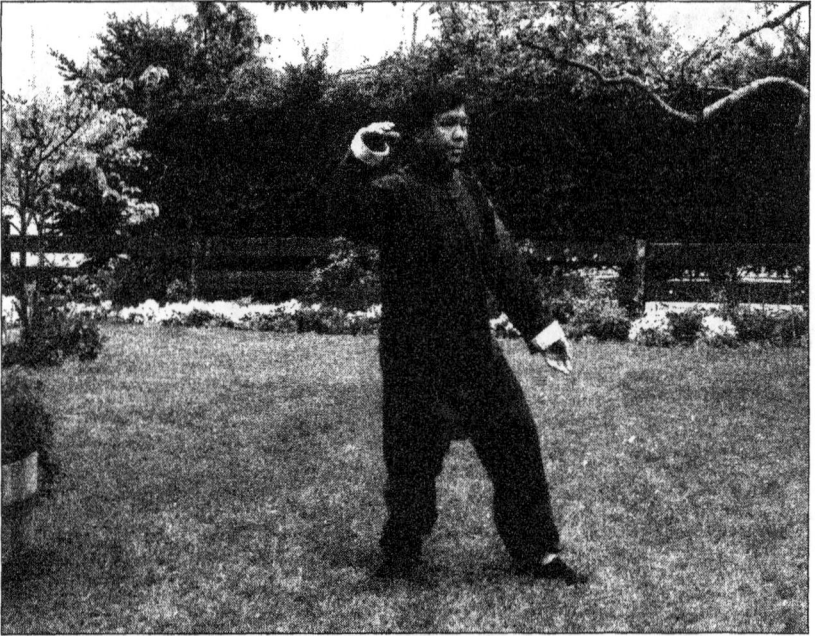

Henry demonstrating tai chi posture *"Brace Tiger Return to Mountain"*

A circle contains immense power. By positioning his body into a circular shape, Henry is able to use his centre and also to remain rooted when students attempt to move him. My experience when pushing against his arm is similar to pressing against a highly inflated rubber ball. The ball metaphor also describes Henry's ability to bounce me off his body, by receiving my force and reflecting it back through my centre. He states it is similar to returning a volley ball.

Just like a ball, the body contains an infinite number of circles. In addition, the body includes many spirals which absorb or express energy, much like a coiled spring. The tighter, more efficient spiral transmits more energy. When I pushed against Henry's arm in the above example, my force was transmitted in a spiral through his centre and into his rear foot. When this force is reflected back to me, it also travels as a spiral through Henry's body.

Henry describes nine joints and how their connection and rotation create proper spirals and circles during tai chi practice. These joints include the spine, hips, knees, ankles, toes, shoulders, elbows, wrists, and fingers. These joints must rotate in a coordinated fashion, not independently. Henry says that the nine joints move like a snake. By connecting the whole body in a spiral, much energy can be expressed. Any blockage at a joint will interrupt the flow of chi energy. Often when I practice my form, I will hear "popping" sounds which indicates my chi is flowing more freely through my joints.

The next principle is COORDINATION. When we walk naturally, we do so in a coordinated fashion. When my right leg swings forward, I balance it with my left arm, and vice versa. Timing is also a factor. I don't move my arm and later my leg, rather they move simultaneously. When I move through the pattern of thirty seven postures, I focus on coordinating my whole body, especially my arms and legs. When I teach beginning students, I notice how they usually move their body parts separately. Often they will turn their trunk, then remember to turn their feet, eventually jerking their arms into final position. Advanced students will move in a flowing fashion, all body parts connected and moving in a coordinated sequence.

Coordination is controlled by the mind. Again turning to nature for examples, Henry describes how a cat catches a mouse, or an eagle circles its prey. The predator is totally focused on its victim. Its mind has already succeeded in catching the mouse before the cat moves. The cat's centre is on the mouse. Every movement of the cat is coordinated and controlled by the mind.

Controlling my mind is very difficult. When I try to meditate, my mind loves to wander far and wide. Trying to coordinate left and right, up and down, or back and forth is also difficult. Coordination also implies that my movements flow at an even rate of speed, and that each posture flows into the next. It should be impossible to tell where one posture ends and the next one begins.

Finally, Henry talks about "extension" arising from coordinated movements. Individual movements must appear to have no end but seem to extend forever. This extension is the result of my mind's intention, directing my body's movement towards infinity and creating a feeling of energy and spirit (shen). In tai chi we strive for a unity of mental intention and physical movement.

The use of mind also involves the sixth principle, CONCENTRATION. Concentration means my mind is focused on a task. One reason for arising early in the morning to practice my form is that my mind is relatively clear at that time. All too often I find my mind wandering from my form to outside concerns. Remembering the seven principles helps me return to my inner work. If I am distracted, I will not benefit from my practice, and my movements will be automatic and lacking in substance.

When I am concentrating fully, external stimuli will not be noticed. Henry suggests we practice in peaceful surroundings, and without music or other interference. He suggests we practice visualizations to enhance our tai chi. Thinking of flowing water, or energy rays being emitted from the dan tien are examples. Henry sometimes imagines that he is practicing on a surface of ice in order to improve his balance. With concentration I can allow the impossible to become possible. I use concentration to experience my chi flowing through and out of my body. Concentration and extension of chi are used in Chinese healing techniques and qi gong exercises. Development of concentration begins with learning the thirty seven positions of the tai chi form and focusing on the seven principles.

The last principle is RELAXATION. Henry is always exhorting us to "fang sung" or relax. Being relaxed is not the same as being loose or flaccid. Lying on a beach or being sloppy from too much alcohol is not tai chi relaxation. Relaxation requires me to focus on areas of tension in my body and send relaxing messages to those places. I must concentrate on being relaxed.

I carry a lot of tension in my body, especially my shoulders and chest. I shudder to think of the energy wasted in maintaining that tension. I like to imagine the energy available to me once I learn to relax. While working, driving, or socializing, I keep telling myself to relax even more. All through the tai chi form relaxation is a priority. The joints must open and close in a relaxed manner.

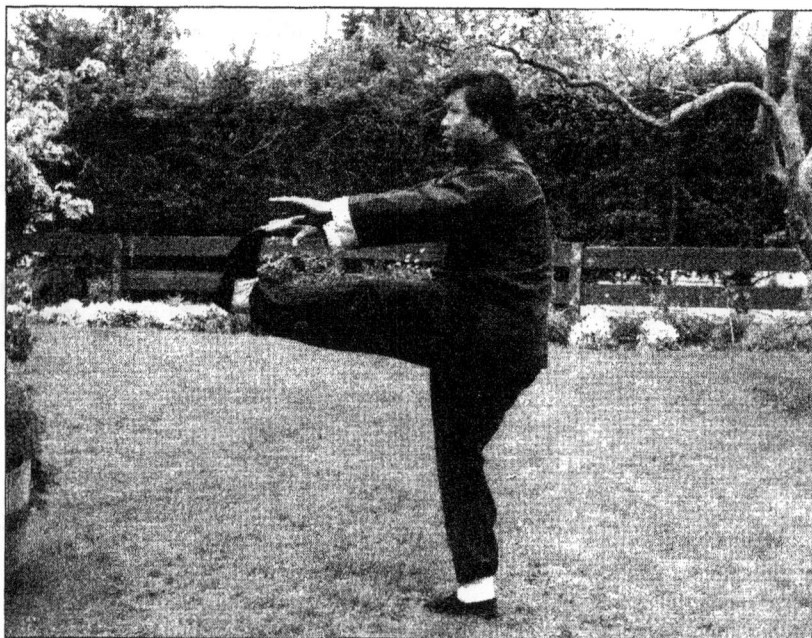

Henry demonstrating tai chi posture "Turning the Body to Sweep the Lotus."

I mentioned earlier the example of bamboo or grass giving way when strong winds blow. This is a natural example of relaxation. Toddlers rarely hurt themselves when they fall because they are still able to be soft. Consider the difference between a rigid lance and a supple bullwhip.

Before practicing my tai chi form I engage in several relaxation exercises to reduce body tension and become softer. Many students are attracted to tai chi solely for relaxation benefits. Henry claims that proper tai chi practice over several years will result in bodily changes. He states our skin will be softer and shinier, and tendons softer and harder to feel. Even bones will increase in density and lose their sharp edges. Our bodies will become less vulnerable to outside shocks. Henry's own body has transformed from tai chi practice. It is hard to feel tendons in his arms, and his bones seem dense. Sometimes he will demonstrate this by letting his arm rest on a student's wrist. The student will experience exquisite pain from the pressure of his arm. Tension causes an arm to feel light. A relaxed arm feels heavy. When shaking Henry's hand, it feels totally soft. Henry can deduce the level of someone's tai chi ability by shaking his or her hand.

So when you see me outside in the morning playing my tai chi form, you will now appreciate how hard I'm working! I am paying attention to increasing details in my movements and applying Henry's seven principles of centre, balance, proportion, circle, coordination, concentration, and relaxation. I need to master these basics in my form and then use the same principles later when I practice search centre. As I realized watching Henry's video, even a master must continue to focus on the fundamental concepts to progress in tai chi.

CHAPTER TEN

Who Studies Tai Chi?

I feel compelled to apologize for that last chapter on the seven principles of tai chi. It is not easy to explain in a book what must be experienced in daily practice. Proper study of the seven principles requires personal discipline and a qualified teacher.

Pretend you want to learn how to ride a bike but have never ridden one. Maybe you have seen a bicycle but never witnessed one being ridden. I will teach you how to ride a bike using the seven principles. First approach the bike and concentrate on the goal of riding down the driveway. Place your body's centre over the seat of the bike, and balance yourself on the bike. You need to place your hands on the handles proportionate to your feet on the pedals. Again focus on each step as it comes, and try to relax. Coordinating your feet, rotate the pedals in a circle, using one hundred percent of your effort on the down stroke and zero percent on the upstroke. (You can attempt to use seventy-thirty weight distribution, but I don't advise it.) You may want to round out your back and shoulders to form a globe shape that is less wind resistant. Continue to focus on these seven principles and off you go. Well, almost.

Yes, I learned how to ride a bike when I was a kid, and I didn't require any principles. Just an older brother and a few bandaids.

Young people seem to be born with certain skills which they lose as they grow older. I mentioned how toddlers are naturally relaxed and rarely hurt themselves when they tumble. As we age, we seem to develop more tension in our bodies and resistance in our lives. Henry rarely has students under the age of twenty five. Younger people prefer body building, competitive sports, or hard style martial arts. Only later do they consider tai chi with its emphasis on softness.

I have found that tai chi practice benefits my other physical activities. I enjoy hiking, cycling, skiing, swimming, and kayaking. When I apply concepts such as circular motion, relaxation, coordination, balance, and movement from my centre, I notice improved performance in these activities. Having chi energy available allows me to engage in fairly strenuous activity such as mountain hiking, without the need to train for weeks ahead.

People study tai chi for many reasons. In Chinese communities, it is part of the culture. Children are exposed to adults performing tai chi in their homes or in the public parks. Most Chinese observe health benefits from daily practice, and also share in the social aspects of meeting others similarly engaged. Probably very few players are serious martial art students.

In North America many non-Chinese have been attracted to tai chi, primarily for health reasons and to manage stress. I am always curious as to why some students decide to continue with tai chi and make it an important part of their lives, while others don't. I have been teaching an introductory course in tai chi for several years at our local recreation centre. Invariably many people sign up for the course, but only a few remain when the course concludes after ten weeks. At first I took this personally but soon realized that most tai chi teachers, including Henry, have similar experiences.

Some students quit their studies, but return at a later time with more commitment. This was my own situation. The beginning classes seem predominantly composed of women or senior citizens, while the advanced classes contain more men and middle aged students. The men seem more attracted to the martial art aspects of tai chi, while women seem content to study the solo form. Of course, these are generalizations, and many exceptions exist. Perhaps the majority of students are content to dabble in tai chi and reach a satisfying level of achievement, while a few become addicted and make tai chi a lifetime challenge.

Henry claims that four requirements are necessary to succeed in tai chi. First a student must be truly interested and dedicated in his/her tai chi practice. Tai chi must become a central part of one's life. I described earlier how Henry sought out many teachers and constantly questioned their teachings. He also was devoted to these teachers in the traditional fashion. He was willing to sacrifice other aspects of his life in order to advance his skills. Many of these choices were not easy for him or his family. The ability to single-mindedly pursue one's life's goals despite family and society expectations may be a trait shared by many great masters in tai chi and other endeavors.

The second requirement is a capable teacher who possesses tai chi skills and the ability to impart them to students.

The third requirement is family support. I have seen many students quit tai chi lessons because it took away from family time. Often their spouses would resent the lack of support with children or household chores. Some family members were jealous of the student's devotion to tai chi or the master. The ideal situation, of course, is when two people can share their interest in tai chi and study together. Ronnie and I are such a pair. Certainly without family agreement and assistance, devoted study is extremely difficult. By leaving Taiwan and moving to Canada, Henry created an environment more conducive to advancing his tai chi. In Canada, life is less demanding and stressful than Taiwan for his entire family, and there are also economic benefits.

The last requirement is sufficient financial support. Many tai chi instructors teach outside the constraints of their regular full time occupation in other fields. This limits their availability to practice and create tai chi. Henry is able to support himself without having other jobs. He has time for research and development of tai chi. Most students do not have this luxury, and therefore their progress is limited. It costs money to take tai chi classes. Henry also has time to integrate tai chi with all that he has learned from other disciplines such as acupuncture, philosophy, calligraphy, herbal medicine, and poetry. His life work requires personal discipline, family support, and financial security.

CHAPTER ELEVEN

Pushing Hands and Butting Heads

After studying a tai chi solo form, many students look forward to the study of "twei shou" or push hands. The practice of push hands involves working with another student, who is termed a partner or an opponent, depending on your point of view. Push hands practice is supposed to develop a student's sensitivity to another person's energy. It also allows a martial application of the principles learned from practicing the solo form.

There are many variations of the push hands concept. Each tai chi style has its own push hands techniques. Basically, however, two partners stand facing each other with one foot forward, divided by an imaginary line on the ground. One player then touches either one or two arms against the other's arm or arms. They then begin a back and forth circular motion while staying in continuous contact through the arms. There are multiple combinations of arm and leg movements taught by different tai chi schools, and some forms of push hands involve moving from the stationary position and stepping backward and forward while still maintaining arm contact.

I don't wish to get lost in describing all the push hands possibilities. I would rather describe why tai chi players do push hands. Theoretically, push hands should teach me to be softer and more sensitive to another's energy. I should be able to sense where in their body they are tense and resistant. By being soft and relaxed, I should be able to use their resistive energy to my advantage and place them off balance. This is accomplished when my partner cannot avoid my advance and has to move his/her position, by lifting a foot

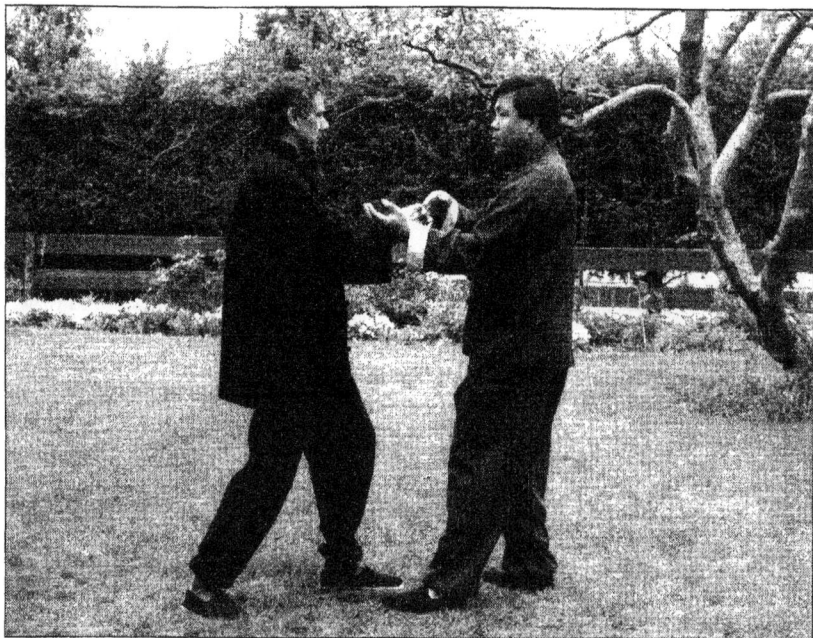

Author and Henry searching centre.

from the ground or falling away from me. I will try to avoid being uprooted myself, by moving softly in a circular spiral away from my partner's arms. The emphasis is on softness and use of energy rather than using force. The Chinese say, "Yung i, bu yung li." (Use mind, don't rely on force.)

That is the theory. What is the practical reality? Until I met Henry, all push hands I encountered involved techniques, tricks, and force. Henry says that the word push in "push hands" already sets the scene for use of muscular force rather than chi. That is why he teaches "search centre," a term which is consistent with a soft style martial art. I will describe search centre in the next chapter. I mentioned earlier that Henry won several push hands competitions in Taiwan. Initially he won by being harder than his opponent. He suffered from pain and bruises for weeks after an event. Later he learned that soft really could defeat hard, just as described in the classical tai chi literature. Four ounces really could move a thousand pounds.

I have watched and participated in push hands competitions and have seen videos teaching push hands methods. Ronnie has attended some of these push hands events and says she can feel the testosterone in the room! It is rare to see two push hands players use softness in competition. The desire to win at all costs takes over, and the result is a lot of shoving, pushing, and grabbing. Players use all kinds of tricks to win. Some push as soon as permissible in order to have the advantage of a first strike. Others depend on wide low stances, or learn to be extremely flexible to avoid being pushed off balance. Many tai chi players avoid competitions because of a realistic fear of being injured. Very few women compete in push hands unless there are separate categories for men and women.

There are lots of rules governing push hands competitions, and these seem to vary with the judges and the event. Points are mainly given for unbalancing an opponent. Occasionally judges will give points for avoiding or neutralizing a push. At a recent competition in Vancouver, the rules gave a player a point if he/she successfully neutralized being pushed, especially if the "pusher" lost his/her balance in the process. Strangely, however, the same event penalized a player who continued to neutralize and not push back. In fact, using too much neutralization was grounds for being disqualified.

Now, my understanding of tai chi is that it is a soft martial art. It is primarily an art of self defence. To me this means avoiding conflicts and not engaging in aggressive acts. In fact, the concept of competition is contrary to tai chi philosophy, in my opinion. What I witnessed in push hands competitions seemed no different than the hard style martial art competitions in the adjacent rings. Why bother learning to be soft when winning competitions depended on being hard? Henry says it is a waste of time to study tai chi if the goal is protecting yourself or injuring another. He claims it makes more sense to buy a gun. I hated competitive sports when I was a youth, mainly because I was a lousy athlete, and usually lost. That may partially explain my dislike for push hands competitions. I don't like the feelings I get when I lose. It's hard for me to let go of that male ego and the desire to win. I don't plan to enter any more push hands events. Henry is organizing search centre events in hopes of encouraging student cooperation and increased skills in utilizing softness. The initial event took place in May, 1996, in Comox, and was very successful. The principles of search centre were discussed and points awarded for softness and yielding. Use of force resulted in loss of points.

True martial artists realize that it is the discipline in learning fighting skills that is important. Actual use of fighting is to be avoided by a true master. Such a master knows his/her ability, but doesn't need to constantly prove it to others. I once interviewed a patient who told me, "Doc, I'm thirty years old and have been in three hundred fights. I only lost three of them." I replied, "I am fifty years old, and have never been in a fight."

It takes a long time and lots of dedicated effort to learn proper soft style techniques. I have been studying with Henry for years but still am unable to really use tai chi for defensive purposes. I still carry too much tension and resistance, and the seven principles are not yet an automatic body response.

SEARCH CENTRE

尋中道

CHAPTER TWELVE

Search Centre

I have written a brief description of push hands, one of the applications of tai chi played with a partner. Henry learned push hands in the traditional fashion and excelled in competitive push hands tournaments in Taiwan. As mentioned, he was disturbed by the pushing and use of force in push hands and wondered how to use chi and softness. "When the student is ready, the teacher will come." Grandmaster Huang Sheng-Shyan was the first to show Henry that soft techniques existed and were superior to hard methods.

Over time Henry observed Grandmaster Huang pushing hands with his students and tried to discover his "secrets." Henry realized that Huang utilized the seven principles though he did not describe or teach them to his students. Huang also used the hundred-zero, and fifty-fifty weight distribution but continued to teach the traditional seventy-thirty concept. I have seen a video in which Huang teaches his students all the traditional concepts of push hands. Yet when he actually engages in push hands, he is using different ideas. This discrepancy makes learning difficult. Many years were required to integrate ideas learned from Huang with Henry's own research and study of tai chi form and push hands. Henry termed the final product "search centre."

Unlike the "push" of push hands, "search centre" gives a softer message and implies the use of sensitivity in finding a partner's centre. To the outside observer search centre may look similar to push hands. Players face each other with one foot forward. One or two hands may be employed, and players move in circles, spiralling from their centres, with arms in soft contact. Hands and arms act as antennae, sensing the partner's centre by feeling any strength or resistance. As one player moves forward, the other moves back and tries by using relaxation to avoid having his/her centre contacted. Then he/she moves forward and tries to find the other player's centre. The softer and more relaxed player's centre is more difficult to find. Any tension will send messages to the partner, letting him/her know where one's centre is located.

There should be comfortable energy between the players, and practice should be enjoyable. This should be a mutual learning experience, where the partners teach each other about search centre, rather than a stressful, competitive atmosphere. No one should be pushed or injured in search centre.

Search centre follows the same seven principles studied in the tai chi solo form. The form is a path to learning search centre, and the two are interdependent. One can't learn search centre without first understanding the form. Also search centre practice will improve one's solo form. The form quiets the mind and body and encourages softness, which is so important in search centre.

During search centre practice the player's body must conform to the seven principles and appear to be circular or "globe shaped." When moving back the weight is distributed one hundred-zero, and fifty-fifty when coming forward. The forward position is never more than fifty-fifty, so the front knee is never ahead of the toes. It is vital to keep oneself centred to be aware of one's partner's centre. Centre is vital for balance, and leaning in any direction is avoided. The body must be in proportion and move in a coordinated manner. The muscles and joints must be soft and relaxed. All movements arise from the centre and are circular. The mind must be focused and concentrated on messages being received through the body. There should be harmony and balance in the to-and-fro movements.

Henry described his creation of search centre principles as a continuing process. Initially he based his ideas on the philosopher, Sun Tze's, "Art of War." "The best commander wins the war without losing a soldier." Henry interpreted this ideal to mean don't depend on superior strength. In his daily tai chi practice he learned to avoid his partner's force and yielded until his body turned like a large ball. He learned to yield to pushes from all possible angles and all degrees of strength. By just learning to receive and yield he became aware of his own centre and areas of resistance. He avoided reacting to his partner's force with strength, frustration, or emotion. His whole body became more sensitive and relaxed. He described pleasure when being pushed as it "built" his centre. He found that his body gradually developed less "shape" and became so soft that his partner would almost feel "sucked" inside Henry's centre.

After learning to receive and yield, Henry began to search for his partner's centre. This involved the use of mind and intention. First he would receive information from his partner's centre. This was experienced by sensing tension and resistance. He would then follow these messages from his partner's centre and use his mind to picture and divide their centre. He would focus his mind to send his chi energy towards his partner's centre, being careful not to under- or over-extend his chi. His body had to be properly proportioned and coordinated. By being soft he could sense his partner's position and direction of movement almost ahead of their conscious intent. As a metaphor he describes carefully feeling the edge of a knife blade to determine sharpness, rather than grabbing it and getting cut. This second phase of skill development emphasizes searching for the centre while avoiding any tendency or desire to push and use muscular force.

After finding a partner's centre, he learned to "cover" it with his chi. Having been "covered" by Henry's energy, I can only describe it as a force field surrounding me. I feel trapped, much like a mouse is trapped before the cat pounces. Though no strength is applied, Henry locks onto my centre and captures me. No matter which direction I turn, I can not escape.

Henry says this ability to surround a partner with chi must be practiced for many years to become automatic. The mind must be used to focus the chi to the smallest centrepoint, much like a magnifying glass focuses the sun's heat to start a fire. After his mind is focused on the centre, chi can be extended in different directions and with different force and timing. Using his mind, he can alter the frequency of chi expression. Thus he can decide to send chi in

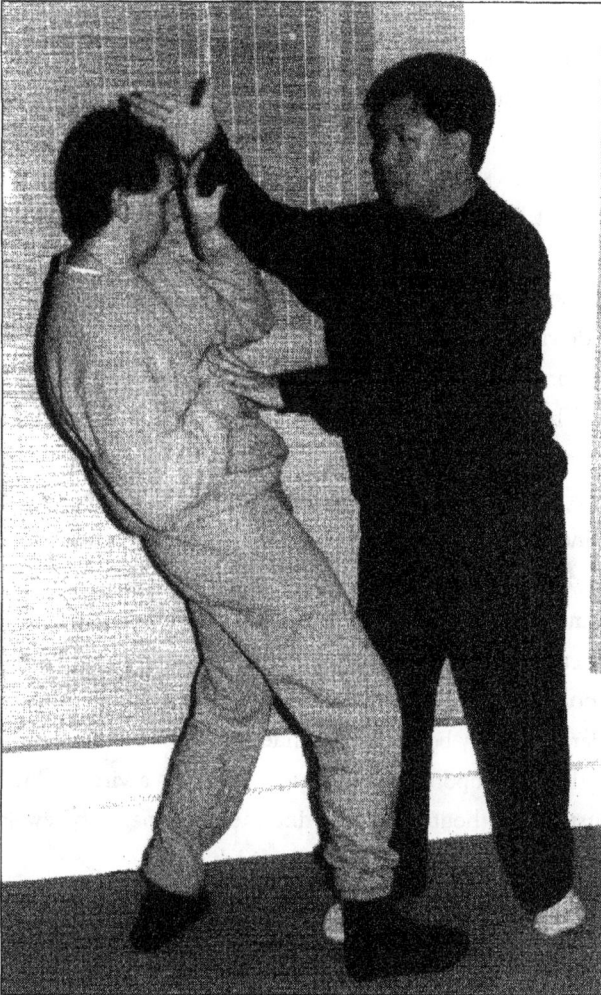

Henry "covering" author.

long slow waves, short fast waves, or some other wave pattern. His chi can be extended from any contact point with the body, such as his shoulder, chest, or back, and not just his hands. The extension of chi past his partner's centre may result in their being moved from their position. This feels like a wind of air or wave of water in its strength and softness. There is no sensation of pain at the point of impact. Depending on Henry's intent, he may cause me to lose my balance only slightly or send me flying across the room. In the latter situation I feel as though I am playing in the ocean surf, and a wave picks me up and moves me down the beach. It's important to note that my body's centre moves first and my arms follow. If Henry had pushed me, the point of contact would move first. The experience is really very pleasurable, and I find myself wanting to do it again.

There is no easy route in learning search centre. It requires years of regular determined practice with players willing to provide constructive feedback. One major difficulty is finding a partner's centre or "chi point," and the direction of its movement. Then when their centre is found, it is not easy for one to remain centred and embody the seven principles. Even with diligent efforts, there are no guarantees one will eventually succeed. Henry realizes that most of his students are only beginning to understand his search centre philosophy. Student attitude is important, and patience really is a virtue. One must practice the first step without contemplating the next one. Very few students are able to achieve, let alone surpass their master's skills.

For the past few years, students have been meeting on Sundays for a drop-in class at a schoolyard in Comox, near Henry's home. There they can get extra practice and instruction in tai chi form or search centre. I can only go infrequently due to the distance from my home and the need to stay overnight. Learning search centre from a fellow student is very different from learning with Henry alone. I find the best approach is a combination with Henry demonstrating on me to allow me to feel what search centre should be, and then practicing with another student with Henry observing and providing critical comments and advice. It is impossible for me to find Henry's centre, but I am able to search a fellow student's.

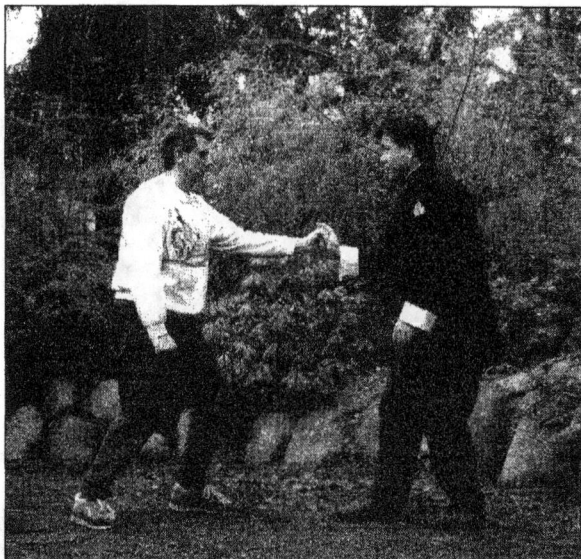

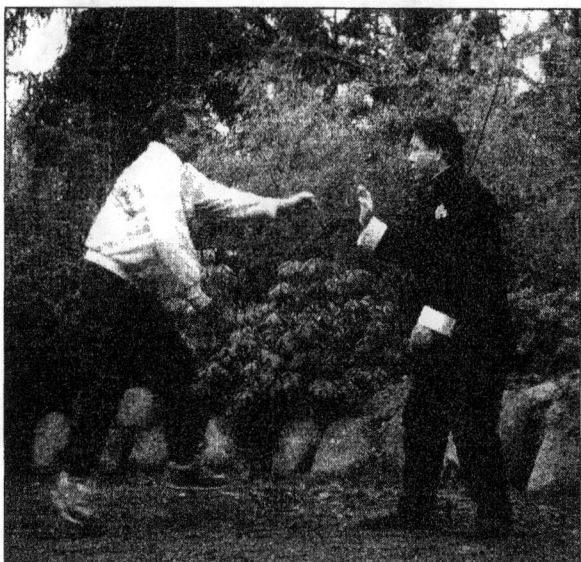

Henry using chi energy to find my centre.

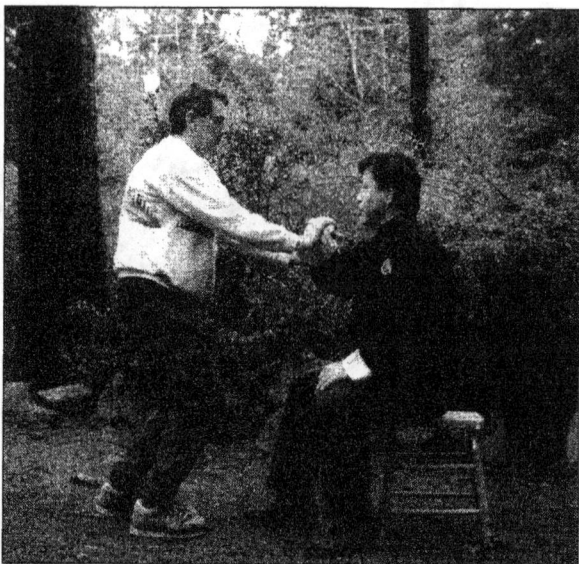

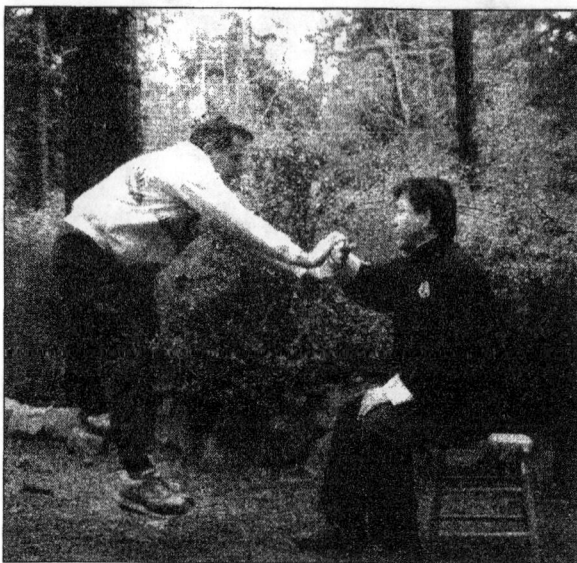

Henry searching my centre without using his legs.

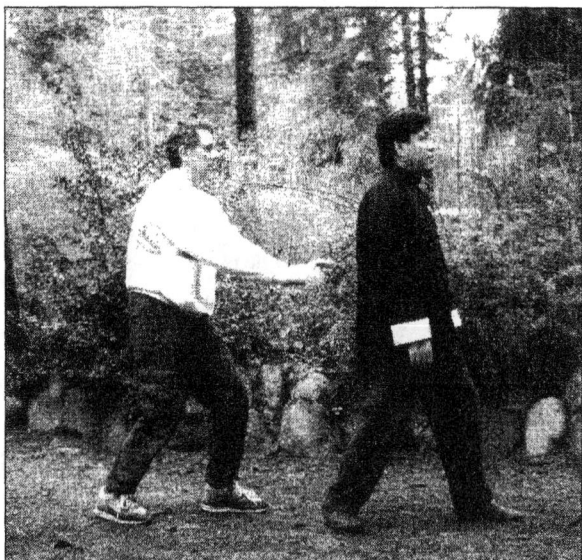

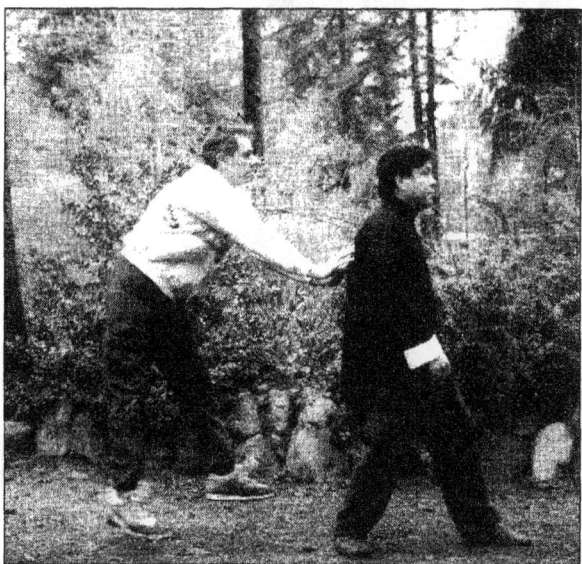

Any part of the body can search centre, even the back.

The practice sessions usually last about two hours. I try to practice with several students since everyone is different. The advanced students in particular can provide important feedback. We try various methods of searching centre. In addition to the most common methods of single or two hand circles, we may try to "root" ourselves while a partner uses force to try to move us. Or we may attempt to throw our partner using only chi energy and avoiding muscular force. One partner will use force to grab or push at various contact points on the body such as arm, shoulder, chest, back, etc. The other partner will try to use search centre principles in each of these situations and "borrow" the force to throw the partner off balance. Henry is always devising new examples to demonstrate the same basic principles.

One of his favourites is having a student grab his little finger. Using only chi energy he redirects the student's force and moves the student off centre. It is not possible to use muscular force in such a situation as a little finger is too weak. We then try to imitate Henry's demonstrations. Each time we practice more is discovered, and technique is refined. I only realize in retrospect how much I have learned. When I am with a beginning student, it is easy to search their centre. With the more advanced students, it is more difficult, but we are able to assist each other and describe what corrections are required. Usually after two hours of practice I am mentally exhausted, while my physical body feels fine, even energized.

I have to concentrate on so many things at the same time to search centre properly. I have to remember to be soft, to initially receive my partner's incoming chi energy, to "lock on to" their centre, to spiral that incoming energy through my body and into the ground. The ability to receive is most important. At first I kept my rear leg tense but only recently understood that my entire body must be relaxed. It feels almost as though my body is a pipe or conduit for the flow of incoming energy, rather than a stiff rod. If I am resisting and don't allow the energy to flow, then muscle tension and pain will be experienced. One advanced student, Edgar, tries to experience his partner's point of contact becoming part of his own body, which he can then move about at will.

Then I must reverse the process. Henry likens it to bouncing a volleyball. My body's tight inner spirals must uncoil in small circles. Then my mind must sense my partner's chi point and focus my outgoing energy from my centre through our mutual point of contact, and extend the energy to a chosen point in the distance. The outgoing energy must come from my centre and not from my arms or body muscles. Chi energy should radiate from my entire body, not just my limbs. There should be minimal body movement. "Bu yung chiao." Don't rely on techniques. Hopefully with practice my search centre skills will become an automatic reflex. Search centre concepts can be applied in all martial arts, including wrestling, judo, or other hard styles. If one really understands search centre principles and can act instinctively, one can theoretically cope with any martial art situation.

Search centre can also be applied to weapons, such as swords, sticks, knives, etc. One of Henry's favourite demonstrations is using something soft such as a rolled up piece of newspaper, or even more dramatic, something fragile such as a long florescent light bulb, in searching a student's centre. In his hands these items become potential weapons. If he used force rather than chi energy, the light bulb would break.

Many of Henry's students have studied other fighting sports and attempt to use them successfully with him. One student uses search centre principles while teaching Kendo, a Japanese martial art. Another student, a policeman, has even tried to use the notorious "choke hold" on Henry. Using search centre principles, he easily escaped, while at the same time placing the student in a vulnerable position. I have yet to witness someone using a fighting technique that Henry can't defend himself against using his search centre ability.

CONCENTRATION

専心一致

CHAPTER THIRTEEN

Search Centre II

I love search centre. In fact it's my second favourite form of physical contact. When Henry lived in our home prior to immigrating, we would practice
search centre every day, sometimes for hours. My body would feel wonderful
after each day's workout. I think I would get "high" physically, from the chi
energy Henry emitted during search centre. I also could feel myself getting
softer and more relaxed. Now that he lives in Comox, I miss the regular search
centre practice.

I think most of Henry's advanced students are captivated by search centre
study. On the one hand it seems so simple and basic when we watch Henry,
while on the other hand it is so frustrating to accomplish on our own. He
makes it look so natural. In class he will put a chair in the middle of the room.
Then he will ask a student to pick up the chair. The student will instinctively
know where to place his hands and how much effort to use in order to pick up
the chair. Henry then smiles and exclaims: "This is search centre!" The student didn't have to think about the process of picking up the chair. Henry
finds my centre in a similar manner, instinctively, but after years of practice.

In Powell River, we tell a story about the large pulp and paper mill. It
seemed that one day it broke down and no machinery would work. Nobody
was able to fix it. The managers called in an outside expert to repair the mill.
The expert walked around the machines for fifteen minutes. Then, taking a
hammer, he hit a spot on one of the machines. Immediately the whole mill was
functioning normally. The managers were extremely pleased and asked the

expert to send them his bill. The bill asked for one thousand dollars. The managers felt this was too expensive for such short work and requested that the bill be itemized. The bill returned from the expert with the following comments: "Hitting the machinery with a hammer, one dollar. Knowing where to hit the machinery, nine hundred and ninety-nine dollars"!

Learning search centre is so intriguing that it becomes an addiction for many students, including me. Henry loves to teach search centre, and his enthusiasm is contagious. While teaching us, he is also practicing and creating new concepts. Having an accomplished master with advanced skills gives us goals to achieve. We realize what is possible if we will continue striving.

I find that most search centre students are men, though, of course, some women also participate. I think men have more difficulty being physically intimate with each other than women do. Perhaps men's fascination with sports, especially "contact sports," is the permission to touch another man's body. Search centre involves significant physical contact and intimacy in a safe environment. Men seem to feel more comfortable practicing with other men. Women prefer to work with other women. Again this probably is related to the intimacy involved in searching for another person's centre. Some students admit they almost feel "violated" when their centre is touched.

For me a lot of psychological "stuff" comes up. Sometimes I am afraid of letting my power out with another person. I hold back from fear that I will incur my partner's displeasure if I find their centre. If I am too capable, they won't like me, is my reasoning. This of course has echoes in my life in other situations. If I am too smart in class the other students will resent me. If I excel at my work, my colleagues will try to destroy me. And so it goes. Therefore, I will often find myself holding back and not fulfilling my potential.

There is also another aspect. What if I search someone's centre and don't find it? What if I let my power out and fail? This is my other fear, the fear of failure. Perhaps my "potential" isn't all that great. What then? Search centre practice triggers all these personal issues, and forces me to do more work on my emotional and spiritual quadrants.

It is also very difficult for me to receive from others . If someone gives me a present, I feel I must pay them back somehow. If someone is kind to me, I feel I owe them something. I act as if I don't really deserve their kindness. I feel I am not good enough. Search centre practice emphasizes receiving energy from another person and neutralizing it before searching for their centre. To really receive energy is very difficult and requires letting go and softness.

Sometimes I feel superior to others, which I'm sure is related to feeling inadequate. My ego takes over and dominates any relationship. Again search centre triggers all these issues. I want to "teach" others who are less skilled and show them how its done. I get upset if someone does it better or catches on more quickly than I. I keep being reminded how much more "letting go" I need to do.

So I persist with my search centre study, learning something valuable every time I practice. Sometimes I ask my kids to practice with me, which they usually resist. Interestingly their friends love to practice with me. How often do teenagers get to push around an adult, and have them beg for more? Practicing with these kids quickly shows me where my jagged edges are!

Henry is hoping to set up search centre tournaments, similar to the May 1996 event, in place of push hands events. Using search centre concepts in contemporary push hands competitions is possible, but difficult. Henry compares it to playing golf with a ping pong ball. In other words one is comparing apples to oranges.

Search centre rules would differ by rewarding softness and ability to neutralize as well as search. Pushing would be penalized. One proposed competition format would take two competitors and designate one offense and the other defense. After three minutes they would reverse roles. Each match would total six minutes in length. The person on offense would be allowed only five seconds to complete a search after initiating it. Offense must search at least every ten seconds, or after completion of three circles with their partner's arms. It would not be permitted to "run out the clock" by circling indefinitely.

Points would be awarded to offense and defense. Yielding and neutralizing a search earns points for defense. Resisting a search with force will earn points for offense. Pushing by offense will earn points for defense. Obviously pushing and resisting are penalized, while sensitivity and relaxation are rewarded. All competitors would have a chance to experience each other and not be quickly eliminated. Henry hopes that search centre competitions as described would encourage the art of tai chi and stimulate a return to the principles of softness and internal energy.

Competitions can be useful in improving tai chi skills. Henry uses the Chinese expression, "shou lien," meaning to improve one's practice by "pruning." A fruit tree is more productive after removing or altering branches or twigs heading in the wrong direction. Similarly, the tree requires many years to grow and develop properly, under the guidance of the grower. Competitions, classes, workshops, and daily practice are a student's medium for tai chi progress.

In the spring of 1995 there was a push hands competition in Vancouver which I entered along with several of Henry's students. Though his students won several of the prizes, including two firsts, the judges were critical. They found it difficult to judge when players were really soft, and not pushing or pulling. They were not convinced that soft could overcome hard, even when they witnessed it.

Henry even demonstrated his search centre ability to the judges after the formal event, which was very uncharacteristic of him. He really hoped that his ideas would be accepted in this greater forum. He asked one student to place an arm between the winner of the competition and Henry himself. The winner was six feet four inches and over two hundred and fifty pounds. He was much larger than Henry. Then Henry and the winner took positions opposing each other, with the other student's arm between them. With almost no visible motion of his body or hands, Henry threw the large winning student halfway across the room without moving the other student's arm in the process. The judges witnessed this event, but later dismissed what they saw as a "trick" between teacher and student. They have not expressed any interest in Henry's ideas. The Chinese have a wonderful proverb, which loosely translated means "seeing the sky from the bottom of a well."

CIRCLE

身形圓滿

CHAPTER FOURTEEN

Teaching and Workshops

Henry leads workshops in Europe and North America. I recently returned from Boise, Idaho where Henry led a tai chi workshop. Paul, one of Henry's advanced students, lives in Idaho and regularly attends Henry's tai chi summer camp at Mt. Washington in Comox. Each year for the past four years, Paul has invited Henry to Boise to lead a workshop for his students. It gives the Idaho students a greater appreciation of tai chi's infinite possibilities and exposure to Paul's master. The workshop took place in an idyllic mountain setting one hour's drive north of Boise. This was the first time I accompanied Henry to Paul's home. Ray, an advanced student and tai chi teacher in Victoria, British Columbia, attended as well. The students really seemed to enjoy all the attention they received from Henry and the senior students. Teaching students really helps me understand tai chi better, and also helps me realize how much I have learned in all my years of study.

In the West we often teach students with positive reinforcement. If they do something well we try to encourage them and give them positive comments. Henry comes from the Chinese school system where students are told how poorly they are doing and how they need to practice harder. He rarely tells me I am doing well. Instead, he points out all my mistakes and shortcomings. He disagrees with western teaching approaches, and feels it provides students with a false sense of accomplishment. His teaching style is often upsetting to students who don't understand its origins. I know it bothered me for a long time, and I still find myself getting frustrated and upset.

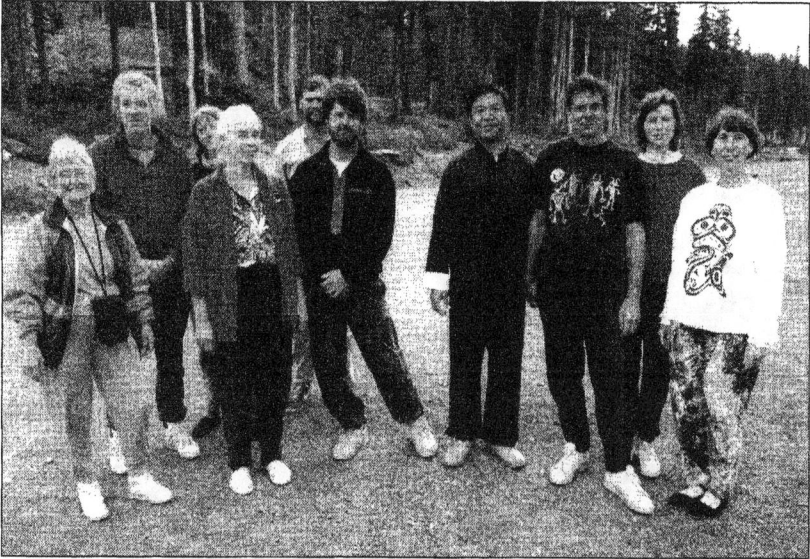

One of the first summer camps at Mt. Washington.

Workshops are an opportunity to learn tai chi with new friends in a comfortable atmosphere. In Idaho a whole weekend was devoted to the workshop. Henry and the advanced students would arise around six in the morning and do exercises and solo form for about an hour and a half. The other workshop participants would watch or follow along as they wished. After breakfast Henry would lead us in form practice until lunch. In the afternoon we studied search centre, which was a totally new concept for most of the junior students. Later we would take a walk or soak in a natural hot spring before supper. In the evening we all discussed tai chi concepts and tried to answer any questions about form, search centre, chi, etc. Henry also demonstrated advanced techniques on senior students, just to give less advanced students some future goals. It's nice to have the luxury of time while learning tai chi.

The annual tai chi highlight is the Mt. Washington summer camp. Now in its ninth year, this event occurs for one week in July. The setting is beautiful. Mt.

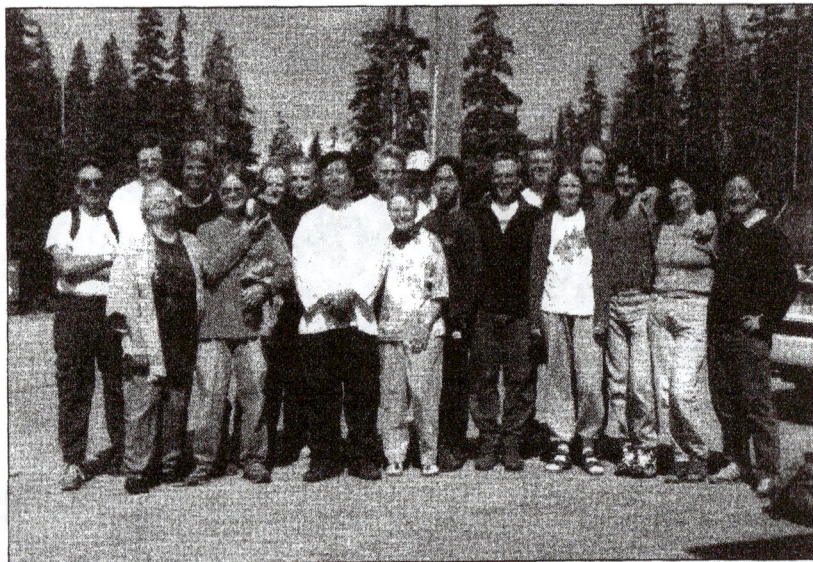

Mt. Washington summer camp, 1997.

Washington is a ski resort in the winter and has chalets for us to stay in. Classes and meals are held at the main ski lodge. We are surrounded by mountain peaks and glaciers, with easy hiking to pristine forests and lakes. The natural chi energy is intense.

Students come from many countries in Europe or Asia as well as Canada and the United States. Some are "regulars" and return year after year. Usually about fifteen students attend. In 1997, there were twenty five. One student, Mr. Hua from Taiwan, had been Henry's student before he moved to Canada. He reunited with Henry at the 1997 camp.

We have a busy day, starting at five thirty in the morning. We practice tai chi meditation under Henry's guidance. This usually involves sitting in a specific posture and breathing from the dan tien. Our minds then meditate on energy flowing in a circle through various important acupuncture points in the head and trunk.

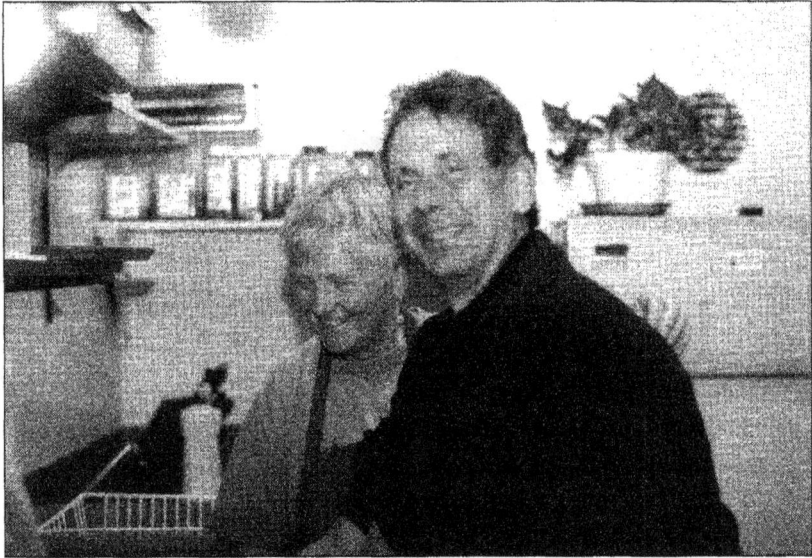

Even the senior students wash dishes at summer camp.

We then walk outside to a flat area overlooking the mountains. There we spend two hours practicing relaxation exercises, qi gong, and form. By the end we are all hungry for breakfast. After eating, we practice the solo form for two hours, often dissecting several postures in minute detail. We will also video ourselves and watch the replay. Finally we spend the hour before lunch studying search centre.

After lunch we rest and then hike to a nearby mountain lake for a swim if the weather permits. Evenings are a chance to practice on our own, watch tai chi videos, and discuss with Henry any aspect of tai chi. It is wonderful to have the input from so many students with various tai chi experiences. For most of us, the intensity of learning in the summer camp provides us with information that will require months of daily practice to assimilate. I enjoy the entire experience and look forward to it each year.

不用技巧

CHAPTER FIFTEEN

Letting Go

Most tai chi players expect major health benefits from studying tai chi. Some even feel that tai chi can prolong life. Certainly Henry is constantly talking about bodily changes resulting from daily practice. He will feel my hands and tell me if my tendons have softened or my bones have become denser. Studies have shown that tai chi can help people with various diseases such as arthritis, hypertension, and stress-related illnesses to name just a few. I recently read that tai chi is used in some treatment centres for alcohol and drug withdrawal.

I have personally experienced improvement in my health from tai chi. For years I have suffered from low back pain. X-rays show degenerative changes in my lower spine from physical trauma. Regular practice of tai chi form and relaxation exercises reduce my back pain and increase flexibility. I still have occassional pain, but it would be worse without tai chi.

I also am able to calm myself during stressful times. If I have to appear in public or am anxious for any reason, I can use my mind to relax myself. One practical application is in the dental chair. When the dentist is working on me, I focus my thinking away from my mouth, and relax my body as much as possible. Sometimes during minor procedures, I prefer to use self relaxation instead of an anesthetic.

Once I was stepping outside my door on a rainy day. The outside deck was wet and slippery. My right foot slipped and shot out from under me while my left foot stayed in the house one step above the deck. I ended up doing a split any ballet dancer would be proud of. I was not injured, however, and picked myself up. Later I tried to reenact the position I had assumed but was unable to get close to it. Henry told me that tai chi can prepare me for an emergency situation and that my body will just respond intuitively. He compares this to the story of a woman able to lift a car when her child is trapped beneath it.

As a psychiatrist and medical doctor, I have advised many patients to study tai chi. Some have complained of joint pains, or musculoskeletal problems. Others have been diagnosed with anxiety or depression. I believe that tai chi can assist in healing these problems, though I caution that regular medical treatments are also required. Chinese traditional medicine teaches that tai chi balances the body's energy and promotes general health.

In the summer of 1994, my greatest lesson in letting go began. I noticed periodic aches on the lower right side of my abdomen. I had never felt anything quite like it, but since it was intermittent I did what any self respecting physician would do. I ignored the symptoms!

Then in September I went hiking in the Stein Valley of British Columbia with my brother, Gary. This was strenuous work as the trails were rocky and steep. My pack was heavy since we carried everything we might need for a week. During the hike, I noticed my groin pain change. It lasted longer and was more annoying. I suddenly realized I was dealing with an inguinal hernia on my right side. I was pissed! Why, when I was active and practiced tai chi regularly, did I sustain a hernia? This was carrying muscle relaxation too far. There was nothing I could do about the situation at the time, so I completed the trip and enjoyed myself.

Upon my return to Powell River I saw our local surgeon who confirmed my suspicions and suggested laparoscopic repair of the hernia. This meant going to the hospital for an operation performed through a metal tube and guided by a video camera. A patch was placed over the hernia, and I was able to go home by the afternoon of the operation. I used tai chi relaxation prior to and after the surgery. I focused on rapid healing and minimal discomfort, and that fortunately occurred. The surgeon told me that all had gone according to plan except that he had to remove a small lymph node that blocked the operative site. He sent the node to Vancouver for pathological examination. I was not worried as I had noticed enlarged lymph nodes all over my body for many years. They started when I contracted infectious mononucleosis in my early twenties, and never completely went away.

A few weeks later I was outside fixing a blockage in my water system when the phone rang. It was my family doctor and good friend. He hesitatingly told me that the report from Vancouver indicated that the lymph node was malignant. I was suffering from malignant lymphoma or a cancer of the lymph nodes. I didn't register much more that he said after that. I told him that I had a water line to fix and that I would talk to him later. I was actually in shock but didn't realize it at the time.

How could this happen to me? Why, when I was such a nice guy and practiced tai chi for years? I didn't beat my wife. I didn't lie or steal. What about all the SOBs that deserve to suffer? I felt that somehow I had failed. I had not done something correctly, and now it was pay back time.

The hardest part for me initially was informing my family. I felt horrible telling my kids, especially. My dad had died from cancer when I was in my twenties, and I didn't want to repeat family history. And what could I tell them? I really had no idea what to expect or what my prognosis was. I still don't. I cried a lot, which helped immensely. Keeping emotions in check was not helpful at all. Everyone around me was loving and supportive. I was amazed at the care and attention I received from friends, colleagues, and patients. In a small town the news spread immediately.

When the initial shock wore off, I considered my options. My lymphoma was slow growing and gave me time to plan. I went to the British Columbia Cancer Institute in Vancouver, where I underwent examinations to determine the extent of my illness. The doctors found more malignant nodes in my neck and suggested a six month course of chemotherapy. Some suggested I could just wait and do nothing until symptoms became apparent, since there was no proof that chemotherapy changed the course of the disease. Since I really had no symptoms, and the disease was found by "accident," this course was a real possibility. Most people felt that it was better to "do something," and I decided to go ahead and be treated. This was accomplished in Powell River with minimal side effects. I was even able to continue working.

My patients were very upset. Those who felt depressed or suicidal hesitated to tell me. They felt guilty that they wanted to die when I had cancer. By working I could deny to myself that I was sick and very scared. I would work all day and then go to the hospital for a treatment. Sometimes while the medicine was being administered through the intravenous tubing, other doctors would come and consult with me about their psychiatric patients. During the six months of chemotherapy I only missed three weeks of work, and two of those were during Christmas. Denial is not just a river in Egypt!

I recently received a computer read-out from the British Columbia medical plan. They monitor physicians' patterns of practice. In 1994, my last full year of work, I saw twice as many patients as the average British Columbia psychiatrist. I performed three times the average number of patient services. I accomplished all of this working only four days a week. The final insult was making $10,000 less than the other psychiatrists. If stress contributes to the etiology of cancer, I was a prime candidate. I really had never considered my work to be so taxing.

When the chemo finished, my cancer went into remission, and my lymph nodes disappeared. I had had six months to reflect on my life. Along with the chemo, I tried alternate medical approaches. With Henry's help I found some Chinese doctors and took their herbal remedies. I still see a Chinese naturopath. But most importantly, I decided to change my life style. I found a psychiatrist willing to work in Powell River, and arranged to quit working completely upon his arrival. After thirty years practicing medicine, including twenty years as a psychiatrist in Powell River I was letting it all go. Once the decision was made, I knew it was the correct one. So did every one else. All who knew me told me I had chosen the correct path.

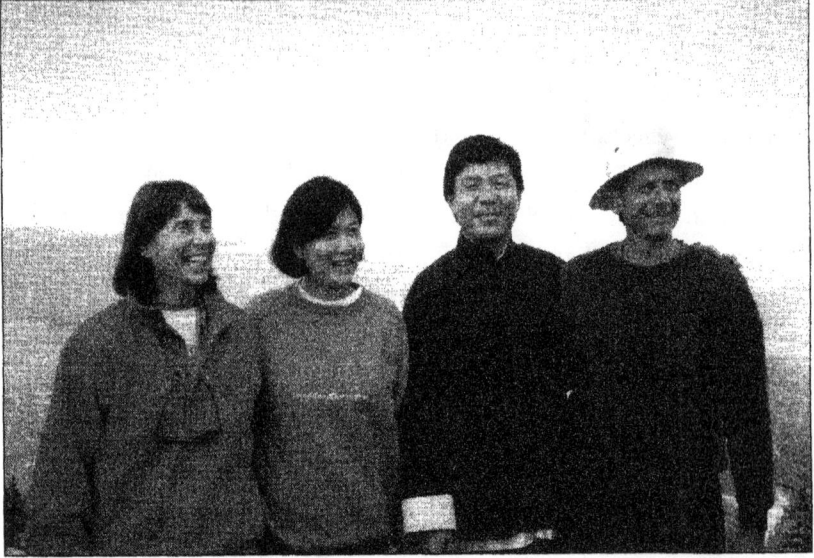

Ronnie, Ivy, Henry and author on top of Mt. Washington, Courtenay, B.C.

It is now over two years since I finished chemo, and two years since I retired. It's been great. I finally have time to do things I never could. I don't know how I ever had time to work. I have time to practice tai chi and visit Henry more often. I decided to write this book. Writing has been another form of tai chi practice for me. I have tried to let my chi energy direct my thoughts and "go with the flow." Henry and I have become more intimate while discussing the book's contents. I hope to teach more.

Most of all I appreciate my life more every day. My relationships with family and friends have taken on a deeper dimension. I am more willing to experiment and do things I would normally be afraid of. My spiritual quadrant is expanding. However, I have my fears of the future. I want to think positively. I want to believe that my cancer is gone and won't return. Its not that easy. When I am alone and honest with myself I realize how frightened I am. I try to cope the best I can with my fears. I am constantly reminding myself to let go.

CHAPTER SIXTEEN

Back to the Future

I have experienced many changes since that day in Riverside Park when Ronnie and I watched tai chi for the first time. I moved from the United States and became a Canadian citizen. Ronnie and I have shared over thirty-five years of marriage, and we have raised three children. We built our own home on forty acres of land in the British Columbia forest and surrounded ourselves with wonderful friends. I have worked almost twenty years as a psychiatrist in an isolated mill town and feel proud of my medical accomplishments. I feel my life has truly been blessed despite my recent diagnosis and treatment. I have greater appreciation for my natural surroundings and the immense love offered to me by family and friends.

Since 1970, tai chi has been a major part of my life. Its influence has fluctuated with other aspects of my life but has always been present. Meeting Henry in 1982 was like getting married to tai chi. My commitment to him and tai chi is almost like a marital bond. He continues to be my tai chi master, my mentor, and my close friend. He has taught me that tai chi is much more than a pretty physical exercise. Through the years we have shared many wonderful and painful life experiences. His philosophy of living in the present, letting go, and loving life has helped me be more accepting of life. I try to control less and enjoy more. I continue to learn more about my body and the possibilities of my mind. Watching him play his form or search my centre teaches me the infinite paths my mind could follow if I only believe and practice. He reminds me that by using my mind "the impossible is possible." I was told by a friend who is a native Salish that white people will believe what they can see. In his culture people will see and experience what they believe.

Henry describes three stages in a student's tai chi progress. The earliest he calls the Jin or energy level. The student is learning the solo form and its various positions or shapes and is beginning to practice the seven principles, especially relaxation. He/she is hoping to achieve a fluidity wherein the movements become connected and individual positions less apparent. Progress will be realized by increased rooting, decreased tension, and bodily changes. The latter may include softening of the skin and tendons, increased muscle flexibility, and a heavy feeling in the shoulders and legs.

The second stage is called the Chi level. The student no longer needs to think about their form in the same way they are able to ride a bicycle automatically. Their form flows freely, and more emphasis is placed on internal feeling. While performing their solo form, they can experience chi flowing through their body. They can practice radiating or extending their chi outside their physical body and develop a sense of a chi "aura" surrounding them. They experience inner warmth, a solid feeling in the dan tien, and tingling in the extremities. The stomach is more relaxed and breathing shifts from the chest to the navel region. The student's form is more related to their internal chi circulation.

The third stage is Shen or spirit. The outside form decreases in importance and the inner spiral predominates. Movement is all in the trunk and centre of the body and the spiral becomes smaller and tighter. Chi flow follows the mind "like water through a pipe," and the form takes on a spiritual quality. Henry talks about seeing a salmon jumping out of the water. He states that the spirit quality of the salmon's leap is just prior to our eyes actually seeing the fish jump. There is spirit immediately before the action. This spirit quality continues during and after the movement. At this stage of development in tai chi, form is almost unnecessary, and movement is all internal. Actions are slow and hard to observe from outside. Bones increase in density, change their shape, and feel softer. Tai chi is integrated in all aspects of one's life, not just one's solo form.

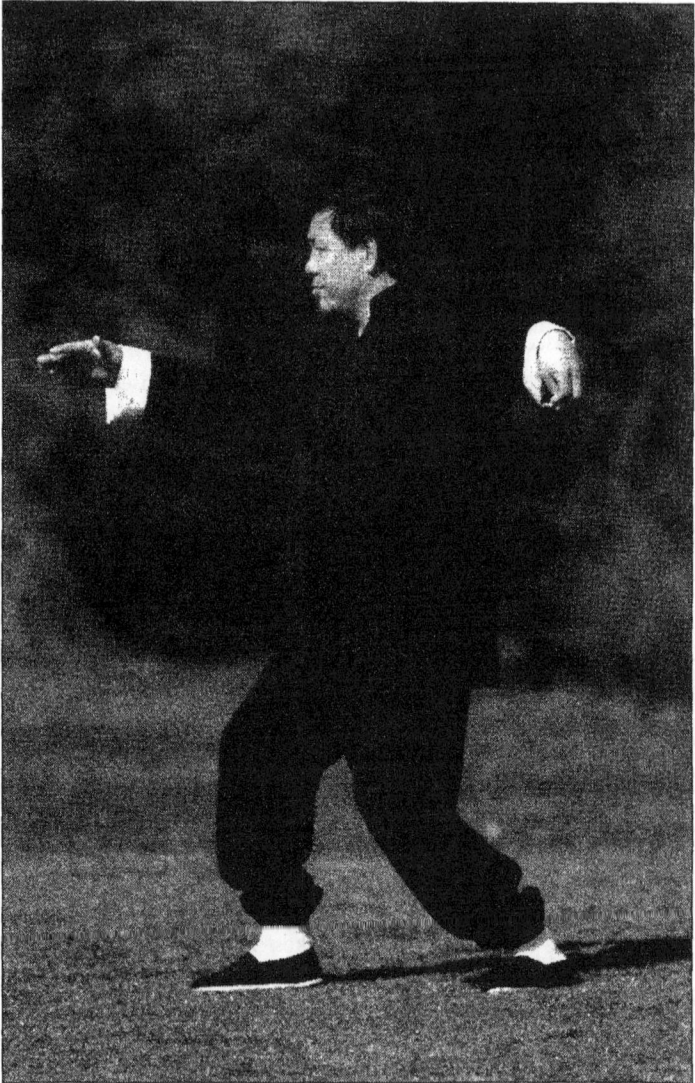

Henry demonstrating tai chi posture "Single Whip."

There is no simple recipe or road map for arriving at these three stages. Many students never reach the higher levels, nor is it absolutely necessary that they do. No specific time periods are required, since all students vary in their abilities. Steady dedicated practice with a qualified teacher and proper attitude are the basic essentials for advancement.

I am not sure where I fit into the above scheme. Perhaps the levels are not so precise, and the borders blend together. My ability seems to fluctuate over time and is influenced by external and internal factors in my life. Besides, there are no "black belts" or official ratings in tai chi. For me tai chi has become **part of who I am** and is not a competitive sport. I try to improve my skills because of the personal benefits that result, not to impress others. I believe the internal work I do for myself will also affect those around me. If I can become centred and peaceful, I can transmit those qualities. By tuning into and receiving the cosmic chi, I can become a transmitter as well.

So I see my future in much the same way as I see my past and present. I will attempt to practice and learn tai chi as long as my life permits. Hopefully my relationship with Henry will continue to bear fruit for many seasons. I will try to use my mind more and attempt the impossible. And I will focus on letting go.

Henry will continue to research and develop creative thinking in tai chi. At the present he is learning how to use his chi from a distance. During search centre practice we sometimes look for our partner's centre without actual physical contact. We are learning to be more sensitive to another's chi energy and respond from a greater distance. To many who watch Henry extend his chi and search a student's centre from afar, it looks fake or at best a trick devised by Henry and the student. They compare it to the children's story of "The Emperor's New Clothes."

Students who have developed sensitivity to energy understand that sending chi from the body is possible. All of us have experienced someone standing or walking by too closely, or "in our space." Sometimes we physically shudder when that occurs. We are feeling their chi. Nobody will argue with massage therapy, but many have trouble with a recent technique called "therapeutic touch" in which healing involves energy fields rather than direct physical contact. I use the analogy of a radio receiver. We are surrounded constantly by radio waves that we are unable to perceive. When we have a radio receiver and turn it on, we are able to connect to the transmissions. It takes time and practice to sense chi transmitted from a distance.

I hope Henry will one day realize his dream of a tai chi "farm." It would be wonderful to have a centre where he can teach and create tai chi with students from around the world. It is not Henry's dream to ever become rich or famous from his tai chi activities, nor is that his concern. He has said many times that people should choose a single path, and his is tai chi. His love for tai chi is apparent in all he does. He has generously brought his love into my life.

CHAPTER SEVENTEEN

Some Suggestions for Improving Your Tai Chi

I mentioned previously that teaching tai chi to less experienced students has greatly improved my own understanding and skills. At first I was reluctant to teach tai chi, because I did not feel adequate to do so. I felt I should have skills comparable to Henry's. He realized that I would learn from teaching others and encouraged me to start my own beginner classes. From observing my students and answering their questions, I have seen common problems which frequently respond to simple corrections. I know when I personally practice tai chi it is impossible to see myself. I may think I am performing a move correctly and it may even "feel" right, but sometimes it's not. Henry or another advanced student can tell me immediately what I need to adjust. If no one is there to watch me, then a video camera can be utilized. In class, Henry will demonstrate one move while two other students attempt to copy him at the same time. The rest of the class then gives feedback to the two students, telling them how their actions differed from Henry's. It's important to provide constructive comments.

In an effort to help students play tai chi better, I will list, in no particular order, some of the frequent concepts that need to be stressed. It is necessary to keep these in mind while practicing daily.

1) Regular practice is vital. I suggest that new students go home after learning a new move and practice that move immediately. If not, the move can be forgotten by the next day. Too many students come to classes unprepared, not having studied between lessons. They then become easily frustrated and quit.

2) Practice in a peaceful place with minimum distractions. Give yourself permission to practice properly and with sufficient time.

3) Focus on the seven principles and understand what they mean. Then practice your form or search centre with the seven principles in mind. It's best to focus on one or two principals at a time and not all of them at once.

4) Use your mind, not just your body. The use of mind in tai chi is its major distinguishing feature from other martial arts. Just learning the movements is not enough. Each action of the body must be directed by the mind. Attention on experiencing and extending chi energy is vital.

5) The trunk and centre always move first. The extremities follow the centre. In every move of the solo form, the body turns first and the arms and legs follow the centre. The body moves as a unit, and there should be a feeling of connection between arms and legs through the body's centre. If arms move independently from the centre, little chi will be experienced, and the movements will appear "external" rather than "internal."

6) Turn your centre, and then shift your weight. Many tai chi schools teach students to shift their position before turning their body. Henry feels this causes imbalance and "double weighting" (where the arm and leg on one side carry the body's weight). In every move, first turn your centre before shifting your weight.

7) When shifting your weight, it is the body's centre that shifts. The centre includes the head, spine, and dan tien. Be careful not to shift weight by leaning the body.

8) The head should be connected to the centre and not move independently. In most moves the head continues to look in the direction of the move and does not turn past a forty-five degree angle. The head faces forward, not up to the sky or down to the ground. Keeping the head over the centre avoids leaning and loss of balance.

9) Muscles should be relaxed. Movements should avoid "pushing." This is especially important in search centre. As long as force is used, expression of chi will be impossible. In search centre the arms act as antennae, sensing a partner's energy. Chi comes from the body and may be transmitted through the arms without the need to push.

10) In search centre practice, learn first to receive a partner's action. Learning to receive and neutralize must be mastered before learning to search another's centre.

11) In searching for another's centre, use softness. Allow your mind to "cover" your partner's centre with your chi. Use your mind to extend your chi through your partner's centre to some point in the distance.

12) When extending your chi in search centre or the form, think of a triangle. The triangle can start from your centre to two points on your partner, and/or from two points on your partner to their centre point. In form practice pick a point far away to direct your chi using the triangle concept.

13) Relate your search centre practice to your study of form and vice versa. Remember that they are interrelated disciplines.

14) Maintain a rounded body shape. Knees and elbows should be slightly bent. Movements follow circles and spirals, not straight lines.

15) Be willing to "invest in loss." If your partner finds your centre, let go rather than resist. Letting go will build your centre.

16) Make sure your weight distribution is either fifty-fifty or one hundred-zero.

17) Remember that all turns are forty-five degrees or multiples thereof.

18) Keep your body level throughout the solo form, especially when turning and shifting your centre.

19) The separate movements in the form should flow together in a fluid sequence. It should be difficult to know where one movement ends and the next one begins.

20) Don't rely on technique in search centre.

21) Study tai chi philosophy.

22) Practice, practice, and practice.

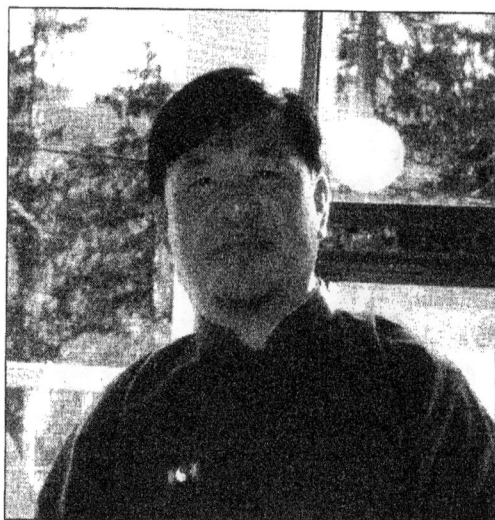

Master Henry Wang

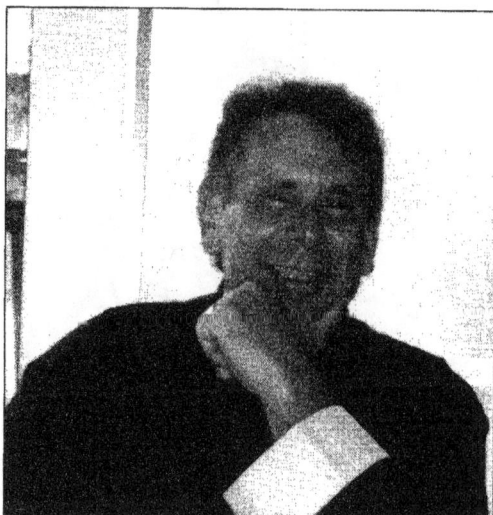

The author, Peter Uhlmann.

Epilogue

I finished writing this book in the spring of 1996. Henry had previously agreed to provide me with some samples of his calligraphy to add to the work. When I visited him at his Comox home he shocked me by saying that not only had he not done the calligraphy, but in addition he did not feel the book was ready for publication. I was devastated as I had worked many long hard hours preparing the book and now he was saying that the time was not right. He tried to explain his position, but I was so upset that none of it really made sense to me.

For years Henry had pressured me to write a book about his tai chi concepts. Until my disability from cancer, I had never had the time. Now the book was almost complete, and he acted as if it was not very important after all. I knew I couldn't argue with him and that he must have good cause to wait. I talked a lot with Ronnie and other senior students, and we all agreed that we would have to delay any book till Henry felt the time was right. Many theories were postulated to explain the situation, but nobody really understood.

I must admit I had a lot of ego tied up in the book. I had already told most of my friends and fellow students that a book was imminent. I felt somewhat foolish all of a sudden, and I was angry at Henry, whom I blamed for my feelings. He had not even read the book but seemed to be acting on his intuition. I worried that the real reason for putting a halt to my writing was Henry's awareness that my understanding of tai chi was too limited and inadequate.

Finally after several months my painful emotions decreased in intensity and life carried on. Little mention was ever made about the book, and it seemed to be history. In the meantime I did publish some articles about Henry and tai chi. I was particularly proud to have an article about the health benefits of tai chi published in the *British Columbia Medical Journal*. After an article about search centre was accepted by *Qi Journal* and another article published about my experience with cancer in the *Canadian Medical Association Journal*, Henry began to compliment me on my writing skills.

In July 1997, I attended the eighth annual tai chi summer camp at Mt. Washington. There were twenty five students, more than in previous years. I began to understand more fully the concepts of search centre at this workshop. Each day seemed to bring more exciting discoveries. For the first time I actually experienced "feeling" someone's centre as opposed to seeing it or thinking about it. Years ago I had asked Henry how he finds someone's centre so easily. He replied that he "felt" it. Now I was accomplishing the same thing, though very crudely. I felt that some hurdles had been jumped, and I was now in new territory.

At the traditional banquet on the last night of summer camp I sat next to Henry and Ivy. At one point in the meal he turned to me and casually mentioned that the time seemed right to publish the book! I couldn't believe my ears. I still don't know what prompted him to change his mind. When I returned to Powell River, I phoned Henry just to confirm what he said. He seemed surprised that I was making such a big deal out of it.

So what was that year's wait all about? I am not really sure. Maybe I never will be. I do know it has been another lesson in "letting go." I also know that my understanding of tai chi increased in that year and is reflected in these pages, particularly the chapters on search centre, which I had to revise. I also learned to trust Henry's intuition and have more faith in my master. Our book is now in your hands.

Song of Section II

Sunshine rising the harbour
I'm going back home
I return to mountain
I rowing my boat
I carry my food
I float in the river
I pass the forest
I see the snake
Crawl up the tree
I see the monkey
Swinging from tree to tree
I open my hand
Stretch out my arm
I follow the bear
Dancing in the circle
I follow the seal
Diving into the water
I learn from the heron
Stand on the rock
I waving to the sky
Learn from the eagle
I waving to the sky
Fly with maple leaf
I turn back a new life
Kick back the memory
I walking in my way
I walking in my way
And return to nature.

MASTER HENRY WANG

www.ingramcontent.com/pod-product-compliance
Lightning Source LLC
Chambersburg PA
CBHW060906280326
41934CB00007B/1211